Pregnancy

DOS AND DON'TS

Pregnancy
DOS AND DON'TS

The Smart Woman's A–Z Pocket Companion
for a Safe and Sound Pregnancy

Elisabeth A. Aron, M.D., F.A.C.O.G.

A Stonesong Press Book

Broadway Books
New York

Broadway Books titles may be purchased for business or promotional use or for special sales. For information, please write to: Special Markets Department, Random House, Inc., 1745 Broadway, New York, NY 10019.

The material presented here is for informational and educational purposes. Although we have attempted to be accurate and up-to-date, some of the contents may become outdated as new information and research become available. Please check with your health care provider if you have any specific questions or concerns.

PRINTED IN THE UNITED STATES OF AMERICA

BROADWAY BOOKS and its logo, a letter B bisected on the diagonal, are trademarks of Random House, Inc.

Visit our Web site at www.broadwaybooks.com

A Stonesong Press Book

Library of Congress Cataloging-in-Publication Data

Aron, Elisabeth A.
Pregnancy dos and don'ts : the smart woman's A-Z pocket companion for a safe and sound pregnancy / by Elisabeth A. Aron.
p. cm.
1. Pregnancy—Popular works. 2. Childbirth—Popular works. I. Title.

RG525.A796 2006
618.2—dc22

2005054225

ISBN 978-0-7679-2089-6

10   9   8

To all the mothers

and

mothers-to-be

CONTENTS

ACKNOWLEDGMENTS

I would like to thank Alison Fargis and everyone at The Stonesong Press for giving me this opportunity and lending their expertise and patience. Writing this book has been an eye-opening experience for me.

Many thanks to all the people who helped to shape my career, but especially everyone at Downtown Women OB/GYN (my old home) and the faculty, residents, and nurses at the University of Colorado Health Sciences Center (my new home).

Thanks to Erica Suchman, Ph.D., at Colorado State University for helping me to understand some of the microbiology of food. Thanks to my head cheerleaders, Bruce and Seth.

Finally, I would also like to acknowledge all the scientists who continue to research issues related to women's health. Having done research for a relatively short time, I can only wonder at all the combined hours spent to obtain this information. Without their continued efforts, we would have no advice to give.

The inspiration for this book came from my pregnant clients, friends, and family members who admitted to feeling crazy with worry about doing practically anything during their pregnancy. We pregnant women are told to avoid *all* drugs, alcohol, certain foods, and beauty treatments, but are not often told what the exact risks are or why we should avoid these things. Further, most physicians (myself included) rarely know the answers to all of your questions without going online or to the library and doing a bit of research.

In an effort to address some of these issues, I have attempted to produce a reassuring guide of what to avoid and what not to worry about during pregnancy. However, while doing the research, I found two very disturbing things: First, not much is known about many of the things we do to our bodies during pregnancy. Second, a lot of reports show associations between various things and bad pregnancy outcomes. These two facts make it very difficult to offer clear advice on questions that have not yet been well researched. I would love to be able to tell you not to worry, but it just isn't that simple. For many issues, providing advice is not black and white.

This book is not meant to be the ultimate and complete guide to dealing with these issues, but a jumping-off point in an effort to educate ourselves and get the answers we need. There may be topics that you are concerned about that are missing. Information about a given topic may change after the publication of this book. This book is meant to help you think about these issues in an intelligent and insight-ful way.

HOW TO USE THIS BOOK

Topics are listed in alphabetical order. I have included icons at the start of each entry to allow for a quick guide as to a product's safety. See page xv for a full description of what the icons represent. However, to really un-derstand the issue, you should read the entire entry.

Each entry has a brief description of the topic followed by any known concerns. The concerns may be legitimate or unfounded and may be based on one small study or on years of research.

"The bottom line" is meant to be the take-home message. When pos-sible, I try to provide a clear answer, but keep in mind that for many top-ics, no clear answer may be available. In this case you must make your own decision. Further, you and your health care provider may not always agree with my opinion; different people have different comfort levels with some of these issues.

Because many pregnant women need to take medications during their pregnancies, I have included many commonly used medications, but it would be impossible to list them all. Most drugs not tested on pregnant women, but their safety during pregnancy is examined by the U.S. Food and Drug Administration (FDA). The FDA looks at information gained from animal testing and other methods and then assigns a risk factor category. See Appendix 1 for a description of what these categories mean. The safest thing to do is to avoid any unnecessary drugs/supple-ments during pregnancy and especially during the first trimester, when the baby's organs are forming. Some drugs are safe in one trimester but need to be avoided in another. Even when the FDA considers a medica-tion safe for use during pregnancy, it is still a smart practice to take drugs only as directed and not to exceed the recommended dosages. This last point goes for everyone, pregnant or not. If you have a question about a medication not listed in this guide, consult your health care provider, your pharmacist, or the *Physician's Desk Reference*. Often this information can be easily found online. Appendix 2 lists many helpful Internet sources.

In cases where the safety of a drug/supplement is not clearly known, I feel that you should educate yourself to understand the risks and benefits. Know the pros and cons when deciding what is right for you during your pregnancy. It is important to understand that not all risks are acceptable to all women, and we must make choices based on what we feel comfortable with as individuals. We should not broadly restrict activities unless there are good reasons or at least some scientific evidence that those activities could cause harm. For example, by understanding the risks associated with eating sushi, I still chose to eat it during my pregnancy because it is less risky than eating improperly prepared or undercooked chicken. Sushi is a great source of protein and omega-3 fatty acids, which appear to help fetal brain development. For me, the pros far outweighed the cons. As long as you understand the risks, you are capable of deciding what is right for your particular situation. If you are not sure about something you've heard or read about, discuss it with your health care provider.

Some pregnancy concerns seem to be overestimated while others have not been publicized enough. For example, even though we all hear that cats carry *Toxoplasmosis*, very few of us know that it is much more common to acquire the disease from undercooked meat or unwashed vegetables. A study in 2001 by the Food Safety and Inspection Service of the U.S. Department of Agriculture determined that many pregnant women were either not aware of the dangers of certain foods or did not handle these foods properly in the home. So while we worry about our litter boxes, most of us are not preparing commonly eaten foods, such as hot dogs and cold cuts, properly and safely.

By limiting your exposure to potentially harmful substances, you can actively work to keep your risks to a minimum while still participating in your regular activities. If you need to work with a potentially hazardous substance, such as paint, limit your exposure by using only the amount needed, by wearing protective clothing, and by using the product in a well-ventilated area. If you do something once or twice during a pregnancy, such as dye your hair, it is unlikely that a brief one-time exposure will result in significant harm. Even so, you can reduce the risks by limiting your exposure, researching the chemicals that are used, and letting your stylist know that you are pregnant.

It is important to use common sense when deciding what is right for you during your pregnancy. It is probably wise to avoid things that are unnecessary and may be potentially dangerous, but at the same time, don't obsess over the things that you cannot control. Although there is no known safe amount of alcohol consumption during pregnancy, don't obsess about the glass of wine you drank before you realized that you were pregnant; it is unlikely to cause any harm to your baby. Moderation in diet, exercise, and work will also help to increase your chances of a healthy pregnancy. No one can guarantee you a healthy pregnancy, but it's comforting to know that you can take some precautions to minimize the risks.

On occasion, a topic includes mention of a specific illness or disease. Appendix 3 briefly describes some illnesses mentioned in the text as well as a few others that you might come across in your reading.

While researching this book, I learned of the many real concerns that exist over the effects of water quality, food quality, and pollutants on our unborn children. We should use these warnings as a wake-up call and work together to try to prevent some of the environmental poisoning that is occurring today. Doing this will help protect all of our futures.

Icons after each entry quickly identify the item's safety. For a full explanation, please read the entire entry. The meanings of the icons are described below and in Appendix 1.

DESCRIPTION OF ICONS

 Dangerous: Known to be dangerous during pregnancy.

 Use with caution: May be dangerous during pregnancy, but may be used if the benefits outweigh the risks.

 Fine: Studies have shown safety.

• • Depends on trimester: May be dangerous if used during certain trimesters and safe during others.

Accutane® *See* Isotretinoin.   ⊘

Acetaminophen   ☑

Acetaminophen, also known as Anacin-3®, Datril®, Panadol®, Tylenol®, and Valorin®, is an over-the-counter pain medication (*see* Pain relievers) and fever reducer. It is an ingredient in numerous cold and flu remedies (*see* Cough and cold suppressants).

CONCERNS: A scientific study noted a link between high (almost every-day) acetaminophen use in the third trimester of pregnancy and wheezing and asthma in children. There was no link with average or high use prior to 20 weeks of pregnancy.

Acetaminophen has been assigned a pregnancy risk factor category of B (*see* Appendix 1). Although controlled studies have not been performed on humans, there is no evidence that taking an occasional acetaminophen or two during pregnancy causes any problems. Further, a prolonged high fever in pregnancy could cause problems for the baby, so you should always try to bring a fever down with acetaminophen.

THE BOTTOM LINE: Acetaminophen is considered to be the safest pain reliever and fever reducer in pregnancy. It is viewed as the pain reliever of choice in pregnancy.

Acidophilus   ☑

Acidophilus is a nutritional supplement that contains the bacteria *Lactobacillus acidophilus*. Many people think that the bacteria aid in digestion and play a role in keeping our immune systems healthy. Acidophilus can be taken orally as a capsule or powder, or is present in some brands of yogurt (*see* Yogurt). It is also available as a vaginal suppository to treat yeast infections.

CONCERNS: Because acidophilus is categorized as a food supplement, it is not regulated by the U.S. Food and Drug Administration. Thus, there is no guarantee of the strength, purity, or safety of this product. If you are experiencing a pregnancy complication, you may want to avoid vaginal suppositories. It is a good idea to inform your health care provider if you are taking any nutritional supplements.

THE BOTTOM LINE: Some studies have observed beneficial digestive effects from taking acidophilus by mouth or using it in a vaginal suppository to treat vaginal yeast infections. Acidophilus may also aid in the treatment of chronic diarrhea; however, its usefulness in other conditions is unclear. Acidophilus appears to be safe in pregnancy.

Acrylic nails

Acrylic nails are artificial nails created by a liquid monomer and a powdered polymer that are combined to form an epoxy. The mixture is then shaped and applied over the natural nail or to a plastic tip that has been glued to the nail. The result is a strong, natural-looking nail that can last for several weeks.

CONCERNS: Because most manicurists find it necessary to wear face masks to avoid breathing in fumes, many pregnant women have concerns about having this treatment and about visiting salons where this treatment is performed. It is also known that some chemicals can be absorbed into the natural nail itself.

No studies have been performed that deal specifically with acrylic nails and pregnancy, but the U.S. Food and Drug Administration has deemed one ingredient used in acrylic nails, methyl-methacrylate (MMA), a health hazard due to the potential of allergic reactions and asthma exacerbations. Be sure to ask your salon if this chemical is used on the premises. Stay clear of any salon that still uses MMA, regardless of pregnancy status. The ingredient ethyl-methacrylate (EMA) is a safer alternative.

THE BOTTOM LINE: If you are worried, avoid the treatment outright while pregnant. Make every effort to limit potential effects by waiting until after the first trimester, when there is less risk to the development of the baby's organs; go to a well-ventilated salon; visit earlier in the day when there are less fumes; consider wearing a mask; and avoid getting chemicals on your skin.

Acupressure

Acupressure is a less invasive form of acupuncture (*see* Acupuncture) that uses thumb or finger pressure, in place of needles, to balance or correct the internal flow of energy. Acupressure has been used to decrease the symptoms of morning sickness, turn breech babies, and reduce labor pains. A typical session can last from 30 minutes to 1 hour.

CONCERNS: Several studies have looked at the effectiveness of acupressure to relieve or reduce symptoms related to morning sickness. Wristband acupressure has been shown to safely relieve or reduce the symptoms of morning sickness. This technique can be applied by a provider, by oneself, or through the use of elastic bands. Some acupoints are thought to help speed or induce labor, and reasonable care must be taken prior to being full term.

THE BOTTOM LINE: Based on recent scientific studies, acupressure does seem to have some usefulness during pregnancy, especially to control nausea. There is no scientific literature indicating that acupressure has been harmful to a pregnancy.

Acupuncture

Acupuncture is based on the traditional Chinese belief that health depends on a balanced flow of life energy, or *qi* (also spelled *chi*). To correct any imbalances, acupuncture needles are placed into acupoints, which act to correct the flow of qi and to redirect the flow of energy to affected areas. Traditional Chinese medicine has used acupuncture for thousands of years to reduce pain during childbirth. More recently, scientific studies have examined the usefulness of acupuncture for infertility, nausea, back pain, carpal tunnel syndrome, turning breech babies, postpartum depression, and the induction of labor.

CONCERNS: Most traditional western OB/GYNs have a limited knowledge of acupuncture and are not likely to recommend its use during pregnancy. Concerns over how it works and the safety of sticking needles into the body have contributed to recommendations to avoid acupuncture during pregnancy. Practitioners of acupuncture caution against overuse throughout pregnancy due to concerns about overstimulation of the fetus. They also suggest avoiding certain acupoints that may stimulate premature labor in the first and second trimesters.

THE BOTTOM LINE: Based on recent scientific studies, acupuncture does seem to have some usefulness during pregnancy, especially to control labor pain, back pain, and nausea, and to increase the success of in vitro fertilization. However, because some acupoints are thought to induce or help speed labor, reasonable care must be taken to avoid these acupoints prior to 37 weeks. There is no scientific literature indicating that acupuncture is harmful during pregnancy. Be sure you visit a licensed or certified acupuncturist. Requirements vary from state to state, but you can learn more through your state's medical board or health department.

Adderall®
Adderall® is a brand name of amphetamine (*see* Amphetamines).

Adrenaline Rush®
Adrenaline Rush® is a brand name of an energy drink (*see* Energy drinks).

Advantage®
Advantage® is a brand name of animal flea medication (*see* Flea and tick medications).

Advil®
Advil® is a brand name of ibuprofen (*see* Ibuprofen; Pain relievers).

Airborne®
Airborne® is a blend of herbal extracts, vitamins, electrolytes, amino acids, and antioxidants. It is used to shorten the duration of the common cold.
CONCERNS: The concerns about the use of Airborne® during pregnancy

are twofold. First, it has been reported that there are about 5,000 inter-national units (1,500 RE) of vitamin A (*see* Vitamin A) in each dose. If Air-borne® is taken as directed, the cumulative dose is higher than the recommended daily allowance (RDA) of vitamin A during pregnancy. If you take several doses as well as your prenatal vitamin you may be at risk for vitamin A toxicity.

Vitamin A is considered to be teratogenic (causing birth defects) in high doses. The U.S. Food and Drug Administration (FDA) has set the rec-ommended daily allowance of preformed vitamin A at 8,000 interna-tional units (2,400 RE) per day during pregnancy. Although no minimum teratogenic doses have yet to be defined, doses of 25,000 IU/day or more are considered to be potentially teratogenic.

The second concern is that this product is considered a food supple-ment and it is not regulated by the FDA. Thus, there is no guarantee of the strength, purity, or safety of this product. You should inform your health care provider if you are taking any nutritional supplements.

Airborne® also contains a small amount of Sucralose (*see* Sucralose; Artificial sweeteners). Small amounts of Sucralose appear to be safe dur-ing pregnancy.

THE BOTTOM LINE: Airborne® is not recommended during pregnancy due to the potential risk of exceeding the maximum recommended daily allowance of vitamin A.

Air conditioners

Air conditioners lower the air temperature in an enclosed area.

CONCERNS: Some people notice increased allergy symptoms when us-ing air conditioners during the summer months, which is often due to nonfunctioning air filters. A simple way to avoid this is to maintain the unit properly. Replace filters according to the manufacturer's sugges-tions; some manufacturers recommend as often as once per month. Air conditioning can also exacerbate the dry skin you may experience during your pregnancy. To help with this condition, consider using a good mois-turizer and humidifier.

There has also been some publicity about the association of Legion-naire's disease outbreaks with air conditioners. Legionnaire's disease is caused by a bacterium called *Legionella pneumophila*, which lives in warm-water environments, such as those found in air conditioners, plumbing systems, and humidifiers. It is estimated that 8,000 to 10,000 people contract Legionnaire's disease every year. However, it is often difficult to diagnose the disease accurately because symptoms can vary from person to person. Unless a doctor specifically suspects Legionnaire's, the appropriate tests are often not performed. The disease is most dangerous to those who have a weakened immune system due to cancer therapy, smoking, or organ transplants. Pregnancy does not appear to be an increased risk factor for getting this disease. While the U.S. Department of Labor's Occupational Safety and Health Administration has standards in place for work-related systems, it is unclear how many cases of Legionnaire's disease are acquired in private homes and what the optimal methods of prevention are. Proper maintenance of all plumbing systems, air-conditioning systems, and humidifiers should minimize your risk of contracting this disease.

THE BOTTOM LINE: A well-maintained air conditioner is safe in pregnancy.

Air fresheners

Air fresheners and aerosol sprays are used to change the odor of the air.
CONCERNS: A recent study examining use of air fresheners and aerosols found an association between their use and an increase in ear infections and diarrhea in young exposed children and an increased risk for maternal depression. The researchers concluded that the cause may have been volatile organic compounds (VOCs). VOCs are a large, diverse group of organic chemicals that exist in a gas form at room temperature. VOCs are found in a variety of materials in the home, including aerosol sprays, new building materials (*see* Building materials), deodorants, and furniture polish (*see* Household cleaners). The majority of VOCs have not been reported to cause any harmful effects, but a few can cause headaches, dizziness, and worsening of respiratory diseases, such as asthma (*see* Asthma). Some VOCs have been recognized to be carcinogenic (cancer causing).

THE BOTTOM LINE: Until more is known about the effects of these household air fresheners, it would be wise to avoid heavy use during pregnancy.

Air purifiers ✓

Air purifiers remove allergens from the air using filters.

CONCERNS: Air purifiers have filters that work to trap particles, such as mold, dust, and pollen, that can cause allergies and asthma (*see* Asthma). When the filter needs to be changed and is not working optimally, these allergens can be released back into the air, causing an allergy or asthma flare-up. A simple way to avoid this is to keep up with the maintenance of your unit. Follow the manufacturer's suggestions for routine maintenance.

THE BOTTOM LINE: A well-maintained air purifier is safe in pregnancy.

Air travel ✓

Air travel involves travel in airplanes.

CONCERNS: People have voiced many concerns and theoretical risks relating to flying during pregnancy, including increased risk of miscarriage; effects of pressure changes, dehydration, noise vibration, and radiation; and increased risk of blood clots at high altitudes.

- *Risk of miscarriage:* One study has shown that flight attendants do have a slightly increased risk of first-trimester miscarriages; however, some researchers now think that the high number of hours a week these women were flying and many other stresses contributed to their increased risk. Similar rates of miscarriage have not been seen in the casual flier.
- *Altitude:* Most commercial airlines keep the cabin pressurized to 5,000 to 8,000 feet (*see* High altitudes). Pregnancy at high altitude has been associated with low birth weight, preterm labor, and preeclampsia (hypertension, protein in the urine, and swelling). However, traveling at this altitude for a relatively short period of time does not appear to cause any pregnancy complications.

- *Dehydration:* Concerns over dehydration are based on an average cabin humidity of less than 25 percent, which is quite dry. However, keeping hydrated is not difficult, and this problem can be overcome.
- *Blood clots:* The theoretical concern that long periods of immobility may cause blood clots to form in the legs has not been substantiated by any published report to date, although much anecdotal evidence exists. Like dehydration, this concern can be easily addressed by moving about or stretching every couple of hours.
- *Noise vibration and radiation:* Studies have shown this is of negligible risk to travelers.

Commercial airlines often require documentation of your due date and may restrict your flight in the third trimester due to concerns that you may deliver in the air. Check with the airline before you make travel plans so you won't run into any unexpected problems. Finally, if you are having a high-risk pregnancy, consult with your health care provider before you travel. Consider taking a copy of your prenatal records with you in case you need emergency care while you are away from home.

THE BOTTOM LINE: Air travel is safe in pregnancy. Obviously, if a complication occurs when you are far from home, you may be forced to deal with new doctors. While traveling, make sure to keep well hydrated and stretch your legs every so often. Seat belt use is encouraged and considered to be safe.

Albuterol

Albuterol is a medication used in the treatment of asthma (*see* Asthma) and preterm labor.

CONCERNS: One study in laboratory mice reports an association between albuterol and an increased incidence of cleft palate. However, no published studies indicate an association between albuterol use and human birth defects. As a result, this drug has been assigned a pregnancy risk factor category of C (*see* Appendix 1). Albuterol can also cause hypotension (low blood pressure) and temporary increases in heart rate and so should be taken with care.

Women with well-controlled asthma have fewer pregnancy complications. In light of this, it seems prudent to take all prescribed asthma medications as directed to keep your asthma under good control. Albuterol may be part of this regimen.

THE BOTTOM LINE: Albuterol is safe in pregnancy.

Alcoholic beverages

Alcoholic beverages are made from a fermented mash of various ingredients, including grains or other plants. Popular types of alcohol include whiskey, gin, rum, vodka, wine, and beer.

CONCERNS: Alcohol is a known teratogen (cause of birth defects). Consumption of alcohol during pregnancy has been associated with intrauterine growth restriction (low birth weight), mental retardation, abnormal facial defects, and other major and minor fetal malformations. Although it appears that fetal alcohol syndrome (FAS) is caused by heavy drinking and/or binge drinking, both the American College of Obstetrics and Gynecology (ACOG) and the U.S. Centers for Disease Control and Prevention (CDC) have stated that no level of alcohol consumption, even the most minimal drinking, during pregnancy has been determined to be safe. A new study found that children who were exposed to alcohol during the first and second trimesters of pregnancy were found to have lower IQ scores. Pregnant women are advised not to drink at all.

THE BOTTOM LINE: Although an occasional sip may be okay, there is absolutely no known amount of alcohol that is safe in pregnancy. Most health care providers recommend avoiding all alcohol during pregnancy.

Aleve®

Aleve® is a brand name of naproxen (*see* Naproxen; Pain relievers).

Allegra®

Allegra® is a brand name of fexofenadine (*see* Fexofenadine; Allergy medications).

Allerest® ☑

Allerest® is a brand name of naphazoline (*see* Naphazoline; Allergy medications).

Allergy medications ☑

Allergy medications are used to treat the symptoms caused by allergies, including nasal itching, runny nose, nasal congestion, watery eyes, and sneezing. Common brands include Allegra® (*see* Fexofenadine), Allerest® (*see* Naphazoline), Claritin® (*see* Loratadine), Nasacort® (*see* Triamcinolone acetonide), and Zyrtec® (*see* Cetrizine). Some are available over the counter while others require a prescription. These medications come in the form of pills, nasal sprays, and eye ointments.

CONCERNS: Most allergy medications have been assigned a risk factor category of B or C (*see* Appendix 1).

THE BOTTOM LINE: Most allergy medicines are considered to be safe in pregnancy. Discuss any specific allergy medications with your health care provider.

Alpha-lipoic acid ⚠

Alpha-lipoic acid (ALA) is a dietary supplement that has been used to treat many conditions, including diabetes, glaucoma, and alcoholic liver damage.

CONCERNS: Since ALA is categorized as a food supplement, it is not regulated by the U.S. Food and Drug Administration. Thus, there is no guarantee of the strength, purity, or safety of this product. Several studies have shown that ALA worked better than placebo in lowering blood sugar.

THE BOTTOM LINE: There is not enough known about the effect of ALA to recommend its use during pregnancy. Diabetes during pregnancy is a high-risk condition and should be treated by a physician with medications that are known to work.

Ambien® ⚠

Ambien® is a brand name for zolpidem (*see* Psychiatric medications).

Amniocentesis

During an amniocentesis, a procedure that is usually performed by an OB/GYN, a needle is placed through the mother's abdomen and uterus into the amniotic fluid cavity to withdraw a small amount of amniotic fluid for analysis. Several things can be determined from the amniotic fluid including signs of infection, fetal chromosomes, and alpha fetoprotein (AFP) levels. Genetic amniocentesis, most often performed at 16–20 weeks, is used to detect certain birth defects, specifically chromosomal abnormalities such as Down's syndrome (trisomy 12) and trisomy 18. Amniocentesis can be performed at other gestational ages to obtain information in the event of a pregnancy complication.

Since amniocentesis is performed for a variety of reasons, you should be fully counseled prior to proceeding. For example, if you are having the amniocentesis to test for Down's syndrome, you should have an idea about what you would do with that information. Some families would want this information to prepare for the child's life while other families may consider terminating the pregnancy if the results were not normal. A second scenario may be testing the fluid for signs of fetal infection in the third trimester. In this case, if an infection were present your physician might suggest an early delivery to minimize the risks to the baby.

CONCERNS: Since amniocentesis is an invasive procedure, the main concern centers on risks of complications from the procedure including risks of miscarriage, damage to the baby, infection, and rupture of membranes. A recent review of over 30,000 amniocentesis procedures done at a single institution showed a pregnancy loss rate of 0.83 percent.

THE BOTTOM LINE: Amniocentesis is not without risk. However, if the benefits outweigh the risks, it may be warranted.

Amoxicillin

Amoxicillin is a penicillin antibiotic (*see* Antibiotics, oral).

CONCERNS: Amoxicillin is an antibiotic that is commonly prescribed in pregnancy. It has been used as part of a multidrug regimen to prolong pregnancy in cases of preterm rupture of membranes and for urinary tract infections. Amoxicillin has been assigned a risk factor category of B (*see* Appendix 1).

THE BOTTOM LINE: Amoxicillin is safe in pregnancy.

Amp®

Amp® is a brand name of an energy drink (*see* Energy drinks).

Amphetamines

Amphetamines are a group of drugs that function as central nervous system stimulants. Brand names include Adderall®, Desoxyn®, and Dexedrine®. They are used for medical conditions such as narcolepsy (a sleep disorder) and attention deficit hyperactivity disorder (ADHD), and as an appetite suppressant. Amphetamines may also be abused by women with substance abuse issues (*see* Drugs of abuse).

CONCERNS: Infants born to women with recent amphetamine use show signs of agitation and can experience withdrawal symptoms. Although no increase in birth defects has been noted with amphetamine use, there does seem to be an increased risk of preterm labor, intrauterine growth restriction (low birth weight), and fetal cerebrovascular events (events relating to the blood vessels of the brain, i.e., strokes). This drug has been assigned a risk factor category of C (*see* Appendix 1).

THE BOTTOM LINE: Illicit or recreational use of amphetamines during pregnancy is not advised. However, if you need to take this medication for a medical condition, you should continue to do so and notify your OB/GYN. With close supervision and monitoring of the baby, the benefits may outweigh the risks.

Amusement park rides

Amusement park rides include Ferris wheels, roller coasters, bumper cars, and bungee jumping (*see* Bungee jumping).

CONCERNS: Disney, Six Flags, Busch Gardens, and even your local state fair may have warning signs not to ride certain rides during pregnancy. The concern with these rides is that sudden starts and stops may be associated with placental abruption (premature separation of the placenta from the uterus). The jarring force from even slow automobile accidents has been shown to cause placental abruption and other complications for women who are pregnant, even when the trauma is not directly to the uterus.

A study of thrill ride injuries in the United States observed that of the 900 million rides taken each year, 1 in 124,000 results in a significant injury. Further, 1 in 15 million rides requires hospitalization and 1 in 150 million rides taken results in a death. Most of the worst injuries are from internal bleeding or from brain damage.

THE BOTTOM LINE: The safest course of action is to avoid amusement park rides that cause jarring during pregnancy.

Anacin®

Anacin® is a brand name for aspirin (*see* Aspirin; Pain relievers).

Anesthetic, local

Local anesthesia is used to numb an area prior to a surgical or dental procedure. Local anesthetic agents are also used for regional anesthesia, such as epidural, spinal, and pudendal blocks. Commonly used local anesthetics include lidocaine and 2-chloroprocaine.

CONCERNS: Toxic effects of local anesthetics are rare but include seizures, hypotension, and cardiac arrhythmias. These risks can be minimized by using only the recommended doses and avoiding injection of drugs into blood vessels.

THE BOTTOM LINE: The use of local anesthetics is safe during pregnancy.

Anesthetic gases, exposure to

Anesthetic gases are commonly used in operating rooms, dental offices, and veterinary clinics (*see* Anesthetic gases, use of). Exposure to gases can occur when working within these environments.

CONCERNS: Studies have shown a possible link between prolonged exposure to anesthetic gases and miscarriage. This is of particular concern to pregnant women who work in hospitals, operating rooms, dental clinics, or veterinary clinics.

THE BOTTOM LINE: Although many of the studies that are quoted are retrospective and were performed prior to increased safety measures, there does appear to be a link between miscarriages and prolonged exposure to anesthetic gases. The U.S. Department of Labor's Occupational Safety and Health Administration has outlined appropriate precautions for workers. Limiting your exposure will help to decrease your risk. Check that your workplace follows these guidelines, and inform your supervisor and human resources office that you are pregnant.

Anesthetic gases, use of ⚠

Anesthetic gases are used to provide general anesthesia during surgeries.

CONCERNS: The use of general anesthesia in pregnant women is associated with serious maternal and fetal complications, including pulmonary aspiration (the inhalation of secretions, food, or water into the lungs) and neonatal depression. One study has shown that fetal exposure of more than eight minutes is associated with increased neonatal depression. Because of this risk, general anesthesia is used only when absolutely necessary, and the use of local anesthetics is encouraged when possible.

There is not enough information on the use of general anesthesia during pregnancy for nonobstetrical procedures. Cases should be individualized, and a team approach involving OB/GYNs, surgeons, and anesthesiologists should be taken.

THE BOTTOM LINE: Although the use of general anesthesia is associated with several serious complications, it is sometimes necessary in certain emergencies.

Antacids ✔

Antacids are used to decrease the amount of acid in the stomach that causes heartburn and gastroesophageal reflux disease (GERD). There are several types of antacids, including over-the-counter and prescription antacids. Some antacids also contain antigas medication (*see* Simethicone). Most antacids are sold over the counter under the brand names of Maalox®, Mylanta®, Rolaids®, and Tums®. Maalox® and Mylanta® are magnesium based; Rolaids® and Tums® are calcium based. Newer medications, classified as proton pump inhibitors (PPIs), act to block secretion of acid from the cells in the stomach and include Nexium® (*see* Esomeprazole), Prevacid® (*see* Lansoprazole), and Prilosec® (*see* Omeprazole).

CONCERNS: The National Resource Defense Council sued the makers of Rolaids®, Tums®, and other antacids, alleging that these products contained harmful levels of lead (*see* Lead), which has been associated with birth defects and learning disabilities. As a result of the settlement of the suit in 1997, the amounts of lead allowable in these products are now strictly regulated.

Calcium-containing antacids are often recommended during pregnancy because pregnancy increases a woman's calcium requirements. Some research has indicated that there may be an acid rebound effect, where the acid content in the stomach increases after taking the antacid, but this is rare. Some people report that calcium supplements cause them to be constipated, so be sure to get enough fiber and water in your diet.

Less is known about the use of newer medications (Nexium®, Prevacid®, and Prilosec®) during pregnancy, but so far they appear to be safe. Until more is known about their potential effects, many physicians recommend avoiding them during pregnancy.

THE BOTTOM LINE: Most antacids are perfectly safe in pregnancy. Most OB/GYNs recommend that you start with one that has calcium so that you get both of the benefits of heartburn relief and calcium for your baby's growing bones. If these are not effective, or if you find you require large doses, consult your health care provider.

Antibiotics, oral ⚠

Oral antibiotics are medications used to treat bacterial infections, such as urinary tract infections (*see* Urinary tract infections), ear infections, or throat infections. If you get one of these common infections during your pregnancy, your health care provider probably will prescribe an oral antibiotic, such as amoxicillin (*see* Amoxicillin), Augmentin® (*see* Augmentin; Clavulanate potassium), Cipro® (*see* Ciprofloxacin), Flagyl® (*see* Metronidazole), Keflex® (*see* Cephalexin), Macrodantin® (*see* Nitrofurantoin), penicillin G (*see* Penicillin), or Zithromax® (*see* Azithromycin).

CONCERNS: Most antibiotics are perfectly safe in pregnancy, but some, such as tetracycline (*see* Tetracycline), should be avoided. Make sure your health care provider knows that you are pregnant and prescribes a drug with a risk factor category of A, B, or C (*see* Appendix 1).

THE BOTTOM LINE: Most antibiotics are perfectly safe in pregnancy.

Antibiotics, topical ⚠

Topical antibiotics are antibiotics in cream or ointment form that can be applied to the skin, mucous membranes, or eyes. These creams and ointments have been used to treat cuts on the skin, acne, and bacterial vaginitis. Some of these products can be purchased over the counter while others require a prescription. Common examples include bacitracin (*see* Bacitracin), Cleocin® (*see* Clindamycin), erythromycin gel (*see* Erythromycin), and Metrogel® vaginal (*see* Metronidazole).

CONCERNS: Most topical antibiotics are perfectly safe in pregnancy, but some should be avoided. Make sure your health care provider knows that you are pregnant and prescribes a drug with a risk factor category of A, B, or C (*see* Appendix 1).

THE BOTTOM LINE: Most topical antibiotics are perfectly safe in pregnancy.

Antifungal medications, oral and topical ☑

Antifungal medications are used to treat fungal infections. Medications can be oral or topical. Common fungal infections include vaginal yeast infections, athlete's foot, and ringworm. A common oral medication used to treat vaginal yeast infections is Diflucan® (*see* Fluconazole). Common topical medications used to treat vaginal yeast infections are Monistat® (*see* Miconazole) and Terazole® (*see* Terconazole).

CONCERNS: Most oral and topical antifungal medications are perfectly safe in pregnancy, but some should be avoided. Make sure your health care provider knows that you are pregnant and prescribes a drug with a risk factor category of A, B, or C (*see* Appendix 1).

THE BOTTOM LINE: Most antifungal medications are perfectly safe in pregnancy.

Antigas medication *See* Simethicone.

Antihistamines

Antihistamines are drugs that act to block histamine, which is the chemical responsible for most allergy (*see* Allergy medicines) and cold (*see* Cough and cold suppressants) symptoms. Some common brand names include Allegra® (*see* Fexofenadine), Claritin® (*see* Loratadine), and Zyrtec® (*see* Cetrizine). Antihistamines are available either over the counter or by prescription.

CONCERNS: Most antihistamines have been assigned a risk factor category of B or C (*see* Appendix 1).

THE BOTTOM LINE: Antihistamines appear to be safe in pregnancy. Discuss individual antihistamines with your health care provider and try to select one that is a risk factor category B.

Antitussives

Antitussives are medications used to suppress coughs (*see* Cough and cold suppressants). They be may sold over the counter or by prescription. Dextromethorphan (*see* Dextromethorphan) is a common over-the-counter antitussive while codeine (*see* Codeine) and hydrocodone often are available by prescription. Common brand names of over-the-counter antitussives include Antituss® and Robitussin®.

CONCERNS: Most antitussives have been assigned a risk factor category of C (*see* Appendix 1).

THE BOTTOM LINE: Antitussives appear to be safe in pregnancy. Discuss individual antitussives with your health care provider.

Anusol®

Anusol® is a brand name for a hemorrhoid medication (*see* Hemorrhoid medications).

Apple cider and sauce

Apple cider is a beverage made by pressing the juice from the apples. It can be served straight or diluted with water. Sweet cider is not fermented. Hard cider is fermented and may contain varying amounts of alcohol. Applesauce is a puree of cooked apples and sugar and may also contain a variety of spices. Apples are an excellent source of Vitamin C, flavonoids, iron, potassium, and magnesium.

CONCERNS: Although there is nothing unsafe about apples and apple products in and of themselves, *Escherichia coli* (*see E. coli* infection) and *Campylobacter* (*see Campylobacter*) bacteria can contaminate unpasteurized apple cider. *E. coli* is a dangerous infection for anyone, but it can even be more serious in pregnancy. Since 1998, the U.S. Food and Drug Administration has required juice labels to document whether the product is pasteurized (*see* Unpasteurized juice) or not. Proper pasteurization, will kill any harmful bacteria and ensure that the food is safe. Hard cider may contain alcohol, which is not recommended during pregnancy (*see* Alcoholic beverages). Applesauce is cooked and does not have the same risks as unpasteurized cider.

THE BOTTOM LINE: Be wary of any unpasteurized food products. Pasteurized cider and juice are perfectly safe in pregnancy. Applesauce, which is cooked, should be safe if stored properly.

Arginine

Arginine is an amino acid that is thought to play a role in healing, the immune system, and the cardiovascular system. Arginine has been used to increase sperm counts and by bodybuilders to promote muscle growth. It is generally consumed in powder form.

CONCERNS: Most people do not need to take this amino acid as a supplement, as they get plenty of it in the normal consumption of meat, poultry, fish, dairy products, and nuts. Some studies have demonstrated that it can possibly help male infertility.

Because arginine is categorized as a food supplement, it is not regulated by the U.S. Food and Drug Administration. Thus, there is no guarantee of the strength, purity, or safety of this product. Inform your health care provider about any nutritional supplements you may be taking.

THE BOTTOM LINE: There is not enough known about arginine to recommend its use during pregnancy.

Artificial coloring

Artificial colorings are added to processed foods to make them appear more appetizing. Artificial coloring is classified as a food additive (*see* Food additives).

CONCERNS: Many artificial colors that were added to foods in the past have been banned in the United States due to their association with cancer. Newer studies have shown that laboratory animals given artificial food coloring demonstrated behavioral disorders. Some researchers have tried to make an association between artificial colorings and attention deficit hyperactivity disorder (ADHD), but that link remains unclear.

THE BOTTOM LINE: It seems wise to avoid food that contains artificial coloring during pregnancy. If present, artificial colorings are listed on all food labels. Small to moderate amounts of food coloring are probably safe in pregnancy.

Artificial sweeteners

Artificial sweeteners are food additives (*see* Food additives) added to processed foods to make the food sweet without adding extra calories. Artificial sweeteners are commonly found in diet sodas and other low-calorie or low-sugar products. Examples of artificial sweeteners include Equal® and NutraSweet® (*see* Aspartame), cyclamate, saccharin (*see* Saccharin), and Splenda® (*see* Sucralose).

CONCERNS: Despite the fact that many pregnant women are told to avoid artificial sweeteners, the U.S. Food and Drug Administration has determined that most artificial sweeteners in foods are safe. Studies have shown that aspartame does not cross the placenta and has not been associated with any adverse pregnancy outcomes. The U.S. FDA also considers sucralose to be safe during pregnancy. Saccharin, on the other hand, is thought to be a low-level carcinogen (cancer causing) and should be avoided, even when not pregnant.

THE BOTTOM LINE: Saccharin should be avoided because of possible links to cancer. Moderate Aspartame and Sucralose intake appears to be safe in pregnancy. Dieting (*see* Dieting) is not recommended during pregnancy, and consequently the use of artificial sweeteners is not necessary.

Asbestos *See* Building materials. ⚠️

Ascorbic acid *See* Vitamin C. ☑️

Aspartame ⚠️

Aspartame, also known by the brands Equal® and NutraSweet®, is an artificial sweetener (*see* Artificial sweeteners) that has no calories. It is found in many sweetened foods, including diet soft drinks.

CONCERNS: Despite the fact that the U.S. FDA declared aspartame safe for use in food in 1981, complaints about this artificial sweetener continue. Aspartame use during pregnancy has been blamed for preterm labor, birth defects, mental retardation, and allergies. Several scientific studies in both laboratory animals and humans have been unable to find any association with birth defects or poor pregnancy outcomes. Aspartame does not readily cross the placenta and is considered to be safe in pregnancy.

One by-product of aspartame that does cross the placenta is phenylalanine. Phenylalanine is dangerous to people with phenylketonuria (PKU), and as a result the FDA requires that food containing this sweetener be labeled as such. Aspartame has a risk factor category of B/C (*see* Appendix 1).

THE BOTTOM LINE: Moderate aspartame ingestion has not been associated with pregnancy complications.

Aspirin ⚠️ ∴

Aspirin is a nonsteroidal anti-inflammatory drug (NSAID) used as a pain reliever (*see* Pain relievers) and fever reducer. Common brands include Anacin® and Bayer®.

CONCERNS: Chronic or high doses of aspirin have been associated with maternal and fetal bleeding disorders and intrauterine growth restriction (low birth weight). Its relation to birth defects is controversial. Low doses of aspirin sometimes are prescribed to pregnant women with an autoimmune disease, such as lupus, and in pregnancies at high risk for hypertension and preeclampsia (hypertension, protein in the urine, and swelling). Aspirin use in the third trimester has been associated with heart defects and should be avoided unless advised by your health care provider.

THE BOTTOM LINE: Aspirin should be avoided during pregnancy, especially in the third trimester, unless specifically recommended by your health care provider.

Asthma

Asthma is a chronic lung condition that is characterized by recurrent airway obstruction. Symptoms of asthma include wheezing and shortness of breath. Many medications are used in the treatment of asthma, including inhalational agents such as albuterol (*see* Albuterol), metaproterenol, and corticosteroids.

CONCERNS: It has been shown that pregnancy does not consistently worsen or improve asthma. Because women with asthma need to use medications on a regular basis, often there is some concern over the effects that these medications can have on the baby. However, most asthma medications are safe in pregnancy, and the National Institutes of Health recommends that pregnant patients be treated as aggressively as nonpregnant patients. Some studies have shown that women with poorly controlled asthma are at an increased risk of having a baby with intrauterine growth restriction (low birth weight). However, closer examination of these studies showed that this was true mainly in a socioeconomically deprived population, indicating the possibility of multiple reasons for low birth weight. It is often difficult to determine the effects a condition/substance has on human health due to the complexities of our lives. Factors such as poor nutrition or tobacco use can make it difficult to interpret study results.

Some women with an acute asthma exacerbation may also require a chest X ray (*see* X rays). Concern over radiation exposure during pregnancy is warranted, but precautions are taken to limit your exposure.

THE BOTTOM LINE: Most asthma medications are safe in pregnancy. Well-controlled asthma may reduce the risk of complications during pregnancy, and medications should be used as directed.

Ativan®

Ativan® is a brand name for lorazepam (see Psychiatric medications).

Augmentin®

Augmentin® is the brand name for the combination of two antibiotics, amoxicillin and clavulanate potassium (see Amoxicillin; Antibiotics, oral; Clavulanate potassium).

CONCERNS: Augmentin® has been assigned a risk factor category of B (see Appendix 1).

THE BOTTOM LINE: Augmentin® is safe to take during pregnancy.

Azithromycin

Azithromycin is an antibiotic commonly used to treat *Chlamydia* and upper respiratory infections (see Antibiotics, oral). Chlamydia (see Appendix 3) is a common sexually transmitted infection.

CONCERNS: Azithromycin has been assigned a risk factor category of B (see Appendix 1).

THE BOTTOM LINE: Azithromycin is safe to take during pregnancy.

Bacitracin

Bacitracin is an antibiotic that is often applied topically (*see* Antibiotics, topical) in the form of an ointment. It is often used for the treatment of skin infections and on cuts and abrasions.

CONCERNS: No association with topical bacitracin use and birth defects or adverse pregnancy outcomes has ever been made. Bacitracin has been assigned a risk factor category of C (*see* Appendix 1).

THE BOTTOM LINE: Bacitracin ointment appears to be safe for use during pregnancy.

Bacteria

Bacteria are unicellular organisms that exist as free-living organisms or as parasites. Most bacteria are harmless, but some can cause disease.

CONCERNS: Most bacteria do not cause disease, but some are responsible for gastrointestinal infections, urinary tract infections (*see* Urinary tract infections), vaginal infections (*see* Bacterial vaginitis), and upper respiratory infections, among others. Many of the illnesses that are caused by bacteria are treated with antibiotics (*see* Antibiotics, oral).

THE BOTTOM LINE: Most bacteria are harmless. Careful hand washing and food preparation can help you avoid many of the bacteria that cause gastrointestinal diseases. By keeping well hydrated and urinating prior to and after sexual intercourse, you may be able to reduce the chance of getting a urinary tract infection. When around others who are sick, wash your hands carefully and avoid touching your face.

Bacterial vaginitis

Bacterial vaginitis (BV) is a common vaginal bacterial infection associated with vaginal discharge and odor. BV is not a true infection, but an overgrowth of the bacteria that normally inhabit the vagina. It is diagnosed by obtaining a sample of the discharge and examining it under a microscope. It is treated by taking the antibiotic metronidazole (*see* Metronidazole).

CONCERNS: Bacterial vaginitis has been associated with preterm labor and preterm rupture of membranes. Due to this fact, most OB/GYNs will screen for this condition and recommend treatment during pregnancy.

THE BOTTOM LINE: Bacterial vaginitis can increase your risk of having preterm labor and should be treated during pregnancy.

Bayer®

Bayer® is a brand name for aspirin (*see* Aspirin; Pain relievers).

Béarnaise sauce

This is a French sauce made from vinegar, wine, tarragon, egg yolks (*see* Eggs), and butter. The eggs are partially cooked and added to the sauce over a double boiler. The sauce may be served with meat, fish, or vegetables.

CONCERNS: Since the eggs are not fully cooked, there is a possibility that they could contain a bacterium called *Salmonella* (*see* Salmonella). *Salmonella* can cause diarrhea, fever, and abdominal pain. It is most dangerous in people who have a weakened immune system. Women who are pregnant do not appear to be at an increased risk of getting *Salmonella*. However, one type of this bacterium can cross the placenta and cause miscarriage, stillbirth, and preterm labor.

Another concern is the wine (*see* Alcoholic beverages) used in the sauce. Fetal alcohol syndrome includes intrauterine growth restriction (low birth weight) and brain abnormalities and is clearly associated with frequent alcohol consumption or binge drinking. Many health care providers recommend that no alcohol be consumed during a pregnancy because it is not clearly known how much alcohol is safe at this time. Since the sauce is not fully cooked, you may be consuming alcohol.

THE BOTTOM LINE: Partially cooked eggs and alcohol should not be consumed during pregnancy. Pasteurized egg products are safe in pregnancy. Cooking eggs to 165°F/74°C will destroy *Salmonella*. Wash your hands and utensils frequently to avoid cross-contamination when cooking with eggs.

Beef

Beef is the meat of an adult bovine (cattle or cow).

CONCERNS: A recent study found a link between high beef consumption in pregnant women and decreased sperm counts in their male offspring. Researchers felt that this was probably not due to the beef itself, but possibly due to the use of hormones, pesticides, and contaminants in the feed that is used in the beef industry. All of these chemicals can become concentrated in the fat cells of the animal. High beef consumption was defined as more than seven beef meals per week.

Properly cooked beef should be safe, but use caution when handling raw beef. According to the U.S. Food and Drug Administration (FDA), roasts and steaks should be cooked to 145°F/63°C and ground beef to 160°F/71°C. Raw and undercooked beef as well as Deli meat (*see* Deli meats, cooked and uncooked; Cutting boards) can become contaminated with parasites and bacteria including *Toxoplasmosis* (*see Toxoplasmosis*), *Listeria* (*see Listeria*), Salmonella (*see* Salmonella), and *Escherichia coli* (*see* E. coli infection).

There have also been some countries, including Britain and Japan, that have banned the sale of beef on the bone due to concerns over the transmission of bovine spongioform encephalopathy (BSE), also known as "mad cow disease," through the bone marrow (*see* Bone marrow).

On the plus side, beef is loaded with protein and iron, both of which are needed for a healthy pregnancy.

THE BOTTOM LINE: Although moderate amounts of beef are probably safe during pregnancy, women who consume high amounts of beef should be careful during pregnancy. Beef that is grass fed without hormones, antibiotics, or supplemented feeds may be a more expensive, but safer alternative. Cooking beef properly will kill all parasites and bacteria. Beef on the bone is considered to be free of BSE in the United States.

Beer

Beer is a low-alcohol (approximately 5 percent) beverage (*see* Alcoholic beverages).

Benzene

Benzene is a colorless, organic solvent used in making plastics and synthetic fibers and in printing, paints (*see* Building materials), and dry cleaning (*see* Dry cleaning).

CONCERNS: Chronic exposure to benzene has been associated with chromosomal abnormalities and cancer. Acute exposure has been associated with central nervous system disorders, anemia, and immune system depression. Benzene can be released into the environment in the form of fumes from the burning of gasoline and into the water supply as a result of spills and from industrial wastes. Benzene can be degraded by some microbes and is unlikely to accumulate in aquatic organisms.

THE BOTTOM LINE: Typical exposure does not seem to cause increased rates of miscarriage or preterm labor. If you need to use benzene-containing products, use in a well-ventilated area and wear protective gear, such as a face mask and/or gloves. Consider having your drinking water tested or use bottled water.

Beta-carotene

Beta-carotene is a precursor to Vitamin A (*see* Vitamin A). It is naturally found in fruits and vegetables. It is also a component of multivitamins (*see* Multivitamins).

CONCERNS: Since beta-carotene is a precursor to Vitamin A, which can cause birth defects in high doses, there has been some concern over using beta-carotene supplements during pregnancy. Although this area is not well studied in pregnancy, women who took up to 30 milligrams a day of beta-carotene did not have any problems.

THE BOTTOM LINE: If you have a well-balanced diet or are taking a multivitamin, it does not seem to be necessary to supplement your diet with beta-carotene during pregnancy. There have been no studies showing that large amounts of beta-carotene lead to toxicity or birth defects.

The Teratology Society has concluded that beta-carotene is not a human teratogen (cause of birth defects).

BHA/BHT

BHA (butylated hydroxyanisole) and BHT (butylated hydroxytoluene) are food additives (*see* Food additives) that are used as preservatives. They are commonly found in foods that contain oils, such as baked products, to prevent the oils from becoming rancid.

CONCERNS: BHA and BHT are on the U.S. Food and Drug Administration's GRAS list (Generally Recognized As Safe). Despite this, these additives have been linked to cancer and fetal abnormalities in animal studies and as a result have been banned in several countries.

THE BOTTOM LINE: Read labels carefully and avoid foods that contain BHA or BHT during your pregnancy.

Biking

Biking is exercise (*see* Exercise) done on a bicycle. The American College of Obstetrics and Gynecology recommends that most pregnant women exercise 30 minutes per day on most days.

CONCERNS: Pregnancy causes your center of gravity to change, which can affect your ability to balance. Most physicians recommend that you abstain from exercise that has a high risk of falling during pregnancy. However, biking on a stationary bike (upright or recumbent) should be fine.

THE BOTTOM LINE: Biking is probably safe in the first and second trimester. However, biking puts you at risk for falling and abdominal trauma and, unless you are using a stationary bike, should probably be avoided as your pregnancy progresses.

Bikini wax

A "bikini wax" refers to the use of hot wax to remove hair in the bikini area.

CONCERNS: Concerns about bikini waxing include worry over the absorption of harmful chemicals and skin infection. These worries seem to be unfounded, as waxing is chemical and drug free. If your skin is sensitive to waxing, it may be best to avoid this type of hair removal during pregnancy.

THE BOTTOM LINE: There is nothing to indicate that waxing, on any part of the body, is unsafe during pregnancy.

Biotin

Biotin is a water-soluble B complex vitamin. It is essential for life, but is synthesized only by bacteria in the intestinal tract, yeast, mold, algae, and some plants. Biotin can be found in yeast, wheat bran, cooked eggs, liver, whole-wheat bread, avocados, and cauliflower. Biotin functions to assist the body in the metabolism of carbohydrates and fats.

CONCERNS: A recent study indicated that as many as 50 percent of pregnant women may be deficient in biotin and that this deficiency may contribute to birth defects. However, further studies are needed to see if these women really had a biotin deficiency or if the results merely reflected a change in metabolism during pregnancy.

THE BOTTOM LINE: Biotin is considered to be safe in pregnancy and does not cause birth defects. It seems reasonable to take a multivitamin (see Multivitamins) that contains biotin during pregnancy or to make sure you get an adequate amount through the foods that you eat. Beyond that, it is too early to recommend further supplementation in pregnancy.

Bismuth subsalicylate

Found in Pepto Bismol®, among other brands, bismuth subsalicylate is used to stop diarrhea.

CONCERNS: This drug causes concern in pregnancy because of the two active ingredients, bismuth and salicylate. In high doses, bismuth has been shown to cause birth defects in sheep. However, no adverse reports in humans could be found for the doses used in commercially available bismuth preparations. Salicylate, also known as aspirin (see Aspirin), has been assigned a risk factor category of C if used in the first and second trimesters and a risk factor category of D when used in the third

trimester (*see* Appendix 1). These concerns are related to the development of bleeding problems in the mother and fetal heart defects.

THE BOTTOM LINE: This is a drug to be avoided during pregnancy. If it
must be taken due to severe diarrhea, it should be taken in the first half
of pregnancy and only in amounts that do not exceed the recommended
dose. Ask your doctor about using an alternative, such as Imodium® (lo-
peramide), which has a risk factor category of B (*see* Appendix 1).

Bisphenol A

Bisphenol A (BPA) is a chemical that is used in the manufacture of plastic beverage containers and in the lining of canned food containers.

CONCERNS: BPA is similar in structure to estrogen, and therefore researchers have speculated that exposure to BPA during pregnancy may
affect the developing fetus. Exposure occurs when the chemical leaches
out into the beverage or food that is held in the container. A recent study
in laboratory rats has shown that exposure to BPA during pregnancy results in an increased rate of breast cancer later in life in the offspring.
Other studies have also shown a possible association between exposure
to BPA and prostate cancer, brain damage and attention deficit hyperactivity disorder (ADHD), Type 2 diabetes, and obesity.

Unfortunately these studies have not been able to be reproduced and
as of yet there is no definitive answer to this question. Currently the U.S.
Environmental Protection Agency (EPA) has set limits on the acceptable
levels of exposure to this chemical and has stated that the amount ingested by the average person is well below this level.

THE BOTTOM LINE: Some research has shown a possible link to breast
cancer, prostate cancer, and brain abnormalities in offspring exposed to
BPA in utero. However, acceptable levels of exposure are not clear at this
time and studies have not been reproducible. Until more is known, use
glass bottles (including baby bottles) as a safer alternative, avoid putting
plastic bottles in the dishwasher as this causes degradation of the plastic and increased leaching of BPA, and throw away reusable plastic bottles that have become cloudy or cracked.

Blue-veined cheese

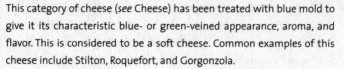

This category of cheese (*see* Cheese) has been treated with blue mold to give it its characteristic blue- or green-veined appearance, aroma, and flavor. This is considered to be a soft cheese. Common examples of this cheese include Stilton, Roquefort, and Gorgonzola.

CONCERNS: Since blue-veined cheese can be made from raw (unpasteurized) milk, caution should be used during pregnancy (*see* Unpasteurized cheeses). All cheese made in the United States is made only from pasteurized milk. The U.S. Food and Drug Administration allows the importation of raw-milk cheese into the United States only if the cheese is aged 60 days or more. The harmful bacteria die as a result of the aging process. Young cheese aged less than 60 days made from unpasteurized milk is not allowed into the country.

Even if the cheese you are eating is made from pasteurized milk, contamination of soft cheese with harmful bacteria such as *Listeria monocytogenes* (*see* Listeria) can occur. This bacterium can cause preterm labor and stillbirth during pregnancy. The Centers for Disease Control and Prevention (CDC) recommends avoiding all soft cheese, including blue-veined cheese, during pregnancy. The high sugar and moisture content of soft cheese is favorable for bacterial growth. The risk of contamination can be decreased, but not prevented, by keeping your refrigerator at 40°F/4.5°C or below; keeping your refrigerator clean; avoiding cross-contamination from countertops, cutting boards, and utensils; and not leaving cheese unrefrigerated for more than two hours.

THE BOTTOM LINE: The CDC recommends avoiding blue-veined cheese during pregnancy. Cooking this cheese until boiling/bubbling should eliminate any harmful bacteria.

Bone marrow

Marrow is a soft, fatty tissue found inside the long bones of animals. It can be cooked inside of the bone or scooped out and cooked separately. It contains mostly fat but has some protein.

CONCERNS: In 1997 the British government issued a ban on the sale of beef (*see* Beef) on the bone after evidence indicated that bones and bone marrow could transmit bovine spongiform encephalopathy (BSE), also known as "mad cow disease." In 2003 Japan followed suit and also banned all meat sold on the bone for the same reason. This action was based on a potential threat of transmitting the disease to humans, but there appears to be very little risk and these bans do not apply to beef bought in the United States.

THE BOTTOM LINE: Bone marrow is considered safe in the United States despite its ban in Britain and Japan.

Boost® energy drink

Boost® is a brand name for a creamy, high-caloric, nutritional drink (*see* Energy drinks).

Botox®

Botox®, also known as botulinum-A toxin, is a toxin derived from the bacterium *Clostridium botulinum*, which is injected into the skin to reduce the appearance of wrinkles. It acts by paralyzing the muscles that cause lines to form.

CONCERNS: Since no studies have been done on pregnant women, dermatologists advise pregnant women not to use Botox® until more information is available to document its safety.

THE BOTTOM LINE: No information regarding the safety of Botox® during pregnancy is available. It is recommended that you avoid this treatment while pregnant until more is learned about its effects.

Bowling *See* Exercise.

Brie

Brie is a cheese (*see* Cheese) that has a white mold rind and a soft, creamy interior. Brie is considered to be a soft cheese.

CONCERNS: Since Brie can be made from raw (unpasteurized) milk, caution should be used during pregnancy (*see* Unpasteurized cheeses). All cheese made in the United States is made only from pasteurized milk. The U.S. Food and Drug Administration allows the importation of raw-milk cheese into the United States only if the cheese is aged 60 days or more. The harmful bacteria die as a result of the aging process. Young cheese aged less than 60 days made from unpasteurized milk is not allowed into the country.

Even if the cheese you are eating is made from pasteurized milk, contamination of soft cheese with harmful bacteria such as *Listeria monocytogenes* (*see* Listeria) can occur. This bacterium can cause preterm labor and stillbirth during pregnancy. The Centers for Disease Control and Prevention (CDC) recommends avoiding all soft cheese, including Brie, during pregnancy. The high sugar and moisture content of soft cheese is favorable for bacterial growth. The risk of contamination can be decreased, but not prevented, by keeping your refrigerator at 40°F/4.5°C or below; keeping your refrigerator clean; avoiding cross-contamination from countertops, cutting boards, and utensils; and not leaving cheese unrefrigerated for more than two hours.

THE BOTTOM LINE: The CDC recommends avoiding Brie during pregnancy. Cooking this cheese until boiling/bubbling should eliminate any harmful bacteria.

Bug spray

See Insect repellents; Insecticides, home use, outdoor use.

Building materials

Building materials include paint, drywall, insulation, adhesives, and spackle.

CONCERNS: Volatile organic compounds (VOCs) are defined as a large diverse group of organic chemicals that exist in a gas form at room temperature. VOCs are found in a variety of materials in the home, including new building materials, paint, varnishes, and carpet. The majority of VOCs have not been reported to cause any harmful effects, but a few can cause headaches, dizziness, and worsening of respiratory diseases like asthma (*see* Asthma). Some VOCs have been recognized to be carcinogenic (cancer causing). While the concentration of VOCs in most homes has been found to be negligible, VOCs can be elevated while painting and using glues. The health effects of VOCs can vary greatly according to the compound, and can range from being highly toxic to having no known health effects. The effects will depend on the nature of the volatile organic compound, the level of exposure, and length of exposure.

- *Paint:* Data are limited regarding the effects of paint fumes (*see* Paint fumes) during pregnancy, and often it is difficult to quantify how much of the chemical is absorbed or inhaled. However, many of the vehicles used to suspend the paint pigments are known to be dangerous. Organic solvents have been associated with an increased rate of miscarriage, cancer, and immune problems (*see* Benzene), and, more recently, lower IQs in offspring from women exposed to organic solvents during pregnancy. Women who have an occupational exposure to paint during pregnancy do not appear to have higher rates of miscarriage. Studies of women who sniffed paint during pregnancy, as a form of recreational drug abuse, showed an increased incidence of children born with features similar to those seen with fetal alcohol syndrome (*see* Alcoholic beverages). Lead can also be found in paint from older homes (*see* Lead) and can be accidentally ingested in the form of dust following sanding or demolition of walls.

- *Drywall:* Most studies examining the effects of occupational exposure to drywall suggest that the greatest risks are associated with physical injuries related to trauma and exacerbation of respiratory conditions such as asthma (*see* Asthma) as a result of exposure to dust during demolition. There is no specific information regarding these products and pregnancy.

- *Insulation:* Potential hazards from using fiberglass insulation result from inhalation of particles and contact with skin and eyes. Fiberglass wool is considered to be a possible carcinogen. There is no specific information regarding these products and pregnancy. Although chronic exposure to asbestos is associated with lung disease (asbestosis) and cancer, short-term oral exposure in laboratory animals has not been associated with any adverse reproductive or developmental effects.

- *Adhesives:* There are limited data on adhesive exposure during pregnancy. Many adhesives contain benzene (*see* Benzene) and other organic solvents that are known to be dangerous during pregnancy.
- *Spackle:* Spackle contains calcium carbonate, magnesium aluminum silicate, and crystalline silica. When sanded, these compounds can take the form of a fine dust and cause eye, respiratory, and nasal irritation. Some of these chemicals are also suspected to be potential carcinogens. The risk appears to be associated with the time and amount of exposure. There are no studies examining their effects during pregnancy.

THE BOTTOM LINE: It appears that many building materials can cause potential health problems, although not many studies involving pregnant women have been performed. If you are sensitive to VOCs or have asthma, use extra care. Some experts recommend delaying any construction projects until after the first trimester to decrease your risk of causing birth defects and avoid using these materials in the last few months of pregnancy or the first few months after birth to avoid risks to the newborn. When using building supplies, try to have good ventilation and appropriate protective clothing to substantially decrease your risks and minimize your exposure to VOCs. If you plan on knocking down a wall, first have the paint checked for lead. If there is lead in the paint, hire someone qualified to deal with this biohazard properly and consider staying somewhere else until the dust clears.

Individual products should be investigated. The National Institutes of Health National Library of Medicine has a database describing known risks of commonly used household products (*see* Appendix 2).

Bungee jumping

Bungee jumping is jumping off a bridge or crane while tethered to a long, strong elastic, or bungee, cord.

CONCERNS: When the bungee cord becomes taut, the jumper rebounds upward. This sudden change of direction shakes both you and the baby, causing some concerns about placental separation as a result of this jerking motion. Although no scientific literature regarding this activity while pregnant could be found, it is safe to say that you should postpone this activity until after delivery.

THE BOTTOM LINE: Bungee cord jumping is not recommended during pregnancy.

Caesar salad ⚠️

This salad is made from romaine lettuce, garlic vinaigrette, Parmesan cheese, croutons, coddled egg (*see* Eggs), and sometimes anchovies.

CONCERNS: Since the eggs are coddled and not fully cooked, there is a possibility that they could contain a bacterium called *Salmonella* (*see Salmonella*). *Salmonella* can cause diarrhea, fever, and abdominal pain. It is most dangerous in people who have a weakened immune system. Women who are pregnant do not appear to be at an increased risk of getting *Salmonella*. However, one type of this bacterium can cross the placenta and cause miscarriage, stillbirth, and preterm labor.

THE BOTTOM LINE: Ask if the dressing contains raw or undercooked eggs. If so, do not eat the salad. Dressings made with pasteurized eggs are fine.

Caffeine ⚠️

Caffeine is an organic compound found in chocolate (*see* Chocolate), coffee (*see* Coffee), cola nuts (*see* Cola nut), and tea (*see* Tea). Caffeine may also be added to cold medicines (*see* Cough and cold suppressants) and energy drinks (*see* Energy drinks). Caffeine is used as a stimulant.

CONCERNS: It is well known that caffeine can stimulate the central nervous system, kidneys, and heart and cause the release of insulin from the pancreas. In 1980 the U.S. Food and Drug Administration (FDA) cautioned women against caffeine use in pregnancy based on animal studies. However, since that time the FDA has amended its initial warning based on research that indicated that moderate caffeine use does not appear to cause birth defects. Some studies have shown that high amounts of caffeine during pregnancy are associated with intrauterine growth restriction (low birth weight). In light of this, most health care providers suggest a reduction in caffeine during pregnancy. If you consume less than 300 milligrams per day, there appears to be little risk. Because amounts differ from food to food, it is difficult to calculate how much caffeine a product contains.

- Coffee can range from 57 to 350 mg per 8-ounce serving.
- Tea ranges from 20 to 110 mg per 8-ounce serving.
- A single (1.5 to 2 ounces) espresso or cappuccino has about 100 mg of caffeine per serving.
- Cola ranges from 30 to 100 mg per 12-ounce can. (The higher caffeine levels are found in "high-energy" colas.)
- A chocolate bar (28 grams) averages 30 mg.
- Cold medicines average 30 mg per dose.

Caffeine has been assigned a risk factor category of B (*see* Appendix 1).

THE BOTTOM LINE: Three hundred mg or less of caffeine per day is safe during pregnancy.

Calcium

Calcium is a mineral that is important for keeping bones strong. During pregnancy, calcium requirements increase from 1,200 to 1,500 milligrams per day. Calcium can be found in dairy products (*see* Cheese), dark leafy green vegetables, soy products (*see* Soy), canned sardines and salmon (*see* Fish), sweet potatoes, and lentils. Calcium can also be taken as a supplement and is a component of multivitamins (*see* Multivitamins).

CONCERNS: If you don't consume enough calcium during your pregnancy, the baby will take its calcium from your bones and put you at risk for osteoporosis. Some studies have linked inadequate calcium intake to an increased risk of developing preeclampsia (hypertension, protein in the urine, and swelling) or gestational hypertension (hypertension related to pregnancy), two serious conditions related to high blood pressure during pregnancy.

Some women report that calcium supplements make them constipated, and calcium can be difficult to absorb. Eating a diet rich in fiber will help prevent constipation, and adding vitamin D can help with calcium absorption.

THE BOTTOM LINE: Make sure you get enough calcium to protect your bones and your baby's development. This can be accomplished by eating three to four servings of calcium-rich foods a day or taking a calcium supplement.

Camembert ⚠

Camembert is a cheese (*see* Cheese) with a white mold rind and a creamy center made from cow's milk. It is considered to be a soft cheese.

CONCERNS: Since Camembert can be made from raw (unpasteurized) milk, caution should be used during pregnancy (*see* Unpasteurized cheese). All cheese made in the United States is made only from pasteurized milk. The U.S. Food and Drug Administration allows the importation of raw-milk cheese into the United States only if the cheese is aged 60 days or more. The harmful bacteria die as a result of the aging process. Young cheese aged less than 60 days made from unpasteurized milk is not allowed into the country.

Even if the cheese you are eating is made from pasteurized milk, contamination of soft cheese with harmful bacteria such as *Listeria monocytogenes* (*see* Listeria) can occur. This bacterium can cause preterm labor and stillbirth during pregnancy. The Centers for Disease Control and Prevention (CDC) recommends avoiding all soft cheese, including Camembert, during pregnancy. The high sugar and moisture content of soft cheese is favorable for bacterial growth. The risk of contamination can be decreased, but not prevented, by keeping your refrigerator at 40°F/4.5°C or below; keeping your refrigerator clean; avoiding cross-contamination from countertops, cutting boards, and utensils; and not leaving cheese unrefrigerated for more than two hours.

THE BOTTOM LINE: The CDC recommends avoiding Camembert during pregnancy. Cooking this cheese until boiling/bubbling should eliminate any harmful bacteria.

Camomile (chamomile) tea ✓

Camomile tea (*see* Herb tea) is made from an infusion of dried camomile flowers. Many people find this tea to have soothing properties, and it has been used to aid sleep, for mouth sores, and for morning sickness.

CONCERNS: Since camomile tea is categorized as a food supplement, it is not regulated by the U.S. Food and Drug Administration (FDA). Thus, there is no guarantee of the strength, purity, or safety of this product. There are several additional concerns surrounding the use of camomile tea during pregnancy. Prescribers of herbs have reported that camomile oil (*see* Essential oils) can be used as a uterine stimulant, so camomile oil should be avoided during pregnancy. There have also been some reports that camomile tea may interact with blood thinners. Taking camomile and iron together may reduce the absorption of iron. This interaction has not been proven with camomile tea, but it has been seen with similar herbal teas.

Despite the above, camomile is on the FDA list of GRAS (generally regarded as safe) ingredients and is viewed as a very beneficial and benign herb. Further, a tea generally has low concentrations of herbs and probably does not cause any significant drug interactions. Oils may be more concentrated and thus have stronger effects.

THE BOTTOM LINE: Camomile tea in moderation appears to be safe in pregnancy.

Campylobacter ⚠

Campylobacter jejuni bacteria (*see* Bacteria) are responsible for a large number of food poisoning and gastroenteritis cases. The most common food sources of these bacteria are undercooked meat and poultry, raw shellfish (*see* Shellfish), and unpasteurized milk and juices (*see* Unpasteurized juice). The bacteria can spread from person to person via inadequate hand washing.

CONCERNS: Although pregnancy does not increase your risk of getting *campylobacter*, some strains can cross the placenta to cause miscarriage, stillbirth, and preterm labor.

THE BOTTOM LINE: Cook all foods to the proper temperatures. Wash hands and utensils carefully after handling raw foods to avoid cross-contamination. Avoid unpasteurized dairy products and juices.

Castor oil ⚠️

Castor oil is used to treat a variety of ailments, including constipation (*see* Laxatives). Castor oil has also been thought to help to ripen the cervix and induce labor at term.

CONCERNS: Studies evaluating the use of castor oil for labor induction have provided mixed results. A few case reports state that using castor oil at term for the induction of labor is associated with serious outcomes, including a uterine rupture, amniotic fluid embolism, and meconium (baby's stool within the amniotic fluid). These events may have been related to castor oil use or may have been coincidental.

THE BOTTOM LINE: Due to its possible association with adverse outcomes, castor oil use to induce labor is not advised. Eating a diet rich in fiber, drinking enough water, and getting exercise (*see* Exercise) should help to prevent constipation and avoid the need for laxatives.

Cat litter *See* Litter boxes. ⚠️

Cats ⚠️

It is estimated that 30 percent of households in the United States have at least one cat. Researchers at the University of Wisconsin in Madison estimate that the total number of pet and free-ranging cats in the United States is more than 100 million.

CONCERNS: Cats that are allowed to go outside can acquire and transmit disease to their owners. One of these diseases, *Toxoplasmosis* (*see Toxoplasmosis*), is caused by a parasite called *Toxoplasmois gondii*. This parasite enters the cat when it eats raw meat (usually birds) and then is passed through its feces. The owner can then acquire the parasite via hand-to-mouth contact after touching the contaminated feces. It is much more common to get *Toxoplasmosis* from eating raw or undercooked meat, from soil that has been visited by infected cats, and from unwashed vegetables. *Toxoplasmosis* can cause fetal death, preterm labor, and birth defects. However, *Toxoplasmosis* is a common childhood infection. Many people are immune to it, and a quick blood test from your health care provider will reveal whether you are immune. If you are immune, there is no need to worry. If you are susceptible, or not immune, you have several options. You can test your cat, keep it indoors, have someone else change the litter pan, or wash your hands very carefully after emptying the litter pan.

Many families are also concerned about how a cat might behave after the arrival of the baby. By allowing your cat time to adjust to the upcoming changes and making sure to give him the attention that he needs, he should adjust nicely. Talk to your vet about any specific concerns that you may have.

THE BOTTOM LINE: Wash hands carefully after changing the cat litter, or, better yet, have someone else do this chore. Talk to your vet about preparing your cat for the baby's arrival.

Cellular phones

Cellular phones, also known as cell phones, are actually sophisticated radios that use low-power transmitters.

CONCERNS: The concern over cellular phones centers on the small electric and magnetic field (EMF) (*see* Electric and magnetic fields) that cell phones produce. Several studies have linked the use of cell phones with certain tumors in laboratory animals. However, no scientific literature has been found that associates cell phones with pregnancy complications. One recent study looked at fetal heart rates via an external fetal monitor during cell phone use and found no changes.

THE BOTTOM LINE: Cell phone use during pregnancy appears to be safe.

Cellular phone towers *See* Cellular phones.

Cephalexin ☑️

Cephalexin, sold under the brand name of Keflex®, is a cephalosporin antibiotic (*see* Antibiotics, oral).

CONCERNS: Cephalexin has been assigned a risk factor category of B (*see* Appendix 1).

THE BOTTOM LINE: Cephalexin is considered to be safe during pregnancy.

Cetrizine ☑️

Cetrizine hydrochloride is an antihistamine (*see* Antihistamines). A brand name for this drug is Zyrtec®. Cetrizine is taken for runny nose and general itching.

CONCERNS: No study has been able to associate cetrizine with any birth defects or adverse pregnancy outcome. As a result, cetrizine has been assigned a risk factor category of B (*see* Appendix 1).

THE BOTTOM LINE: Cetrizine is safe to take during pregnancy.

Cheese ⚠️

Cheese is made from cow, sheep, buffalo, or goat's milk. Some cheeses are pasteurized, a process in which dairy products are heated to kill harmful bacteria, while some are not (*see* Unpasteurized cheeses). Cheese can be further classified as hard, semifirm, semisoft, or soft-ripened. Hard cheeses (parmesan and pecorino) are cooked and aged for long periods. Semifirm (cheddar, Swiss, and Edam) are firm but not crumbly and are cooked and aged, but not as long as hard. Semisoft (Monterey jack, Gouda) may be cooked or uncooked, and soft-ripened cheeses such as Brie (*see* Brie) and Camembert (*see* Camembert) are uncooked.

CONCERNS: Unpasteurized cheese may contain potentially harmful bacteria (*see* Bacteria). These bacteria include *Listeria monocytogenes* (*see* Listeria) and *Campylobacter* (*see* Campylobacter). Pregnant women are 20 times more likely to get *Listeria* than other healthy adults. Infected pregnant women may have symptoms similar to the flu, such as fever and muscle aches, and infection may lead to preterm labor and even stillbirth. All cheese made in the United States is made only from pasteurized milk. The U.S. Food and Drug Administration allows the importation of raw-milk cheese into the United States only if the cheese is aged 60 days or more. The harmful bacteria die as a result of the aging process. Young cheese aged less than 60 days made from unpasteurized milk is not allowed into the country.

Even if the cheese you are eating is made from pasteurized milk, contamination of soft cheese with harmful bacteria such as *Listeria monocytogenes* can occur. The Centers for Disease Control and Prevention (CDC) recommends avoiding all soft cheeses, including feta (*see* Feta), Brie (*see* Brie), Camembert (*see* Camembert), blue-veined cheeses (*see* Blue-veined cheese), and Mexican-style cheeses (*see* Mexican-style cheese), while pregnant. The high sugar and moisture content of soft cheese is favorable for bacterial growth. The risk of contamination can be decreased, but not prevented, by keeping your refrigerator at 40°F/4.5°C or below; keeping your refrigerator clean; avoiding cross-contamination from countertops, cutting boards, and utensils; and not leaving cheese unrefrigerated for more than two hours.

THE BOTTOM LINE: The CDC recommends avoiding soft cheeses during pregnancy. Cooking these cheeses until boiling/bubbling should eliminate any harmful bacteria. All hard, semifirm, and semisoft cheeses are considered safe during pregnancy.

Chewing tobacco

Chewing tobacco, also called "smokeless" tobacco, is placed and held in the mouth to allow for absorption of nicotine through the oral mucosa.

CONCERNS: Tobacco is considered to be a carcinogen and is responsible for many cancers. Several new studies have looked at chewing tobacco during pregnancy. These studies revealed an association between chewing tobacco and decreased birth weight, preterm delivery, and preeclampsia (hypertension, protein in the urine, and swelling).

THE BOTTOM LINE: All forms of tobacco should be avoided during pregnancy. Chewing tobacco is not a safe alternative to cigarettes during pregnancy and may even be more harmful.

Chiropractic treatment ☑️

Chiropractic treatments involve diagnosing spinal misalignments and correcting them using the provider's hands to manipulate or adjust the spine, joints, and muscles.

CONCERNS: Although many women are turning to complementary and alternative medicine (CAM) over traditional western medicine, most physicians in the United States have little experience with CAM and are reluctant to endorse it due to the limited amount of scientific research that has looked at its safety and efficacy. However, a 2006 retrospective study looked at pregnant women who underwent spinal manipulation for pregnancy-related back pain and found that the treatment did not cause any adverse pregnancy outcomes and might have reduced the back pain that these women experienced.

THE BOTTOM LINE: No adverse pregnancy outcomes have been associated with chiropractic treatment during pregnancy.

Chlorine ⚠️

Chlorine is a chemical used to kill harmful bacteria in drinking and pool water.

CONCERNS: A few studies have found that a group of by-products of chlorine, trihalomethane (THMs), can be found in water treated with chlorine and is associated with low birth weight and fetal birth defects, such as neural tube defects. Other studies have not found this association. THMs can be absorbed by drinking or through the skin and lungs. It is unclear what levels are dangerous during pregnancy. Chlorine can also break down into chloroform, which may also cause harm during pregnancy. The Environmental Protection Agency (EPA) has set up standards to monitor these levels and is continuing to do research on this issue.

THE BOTTOM LINE: Until more is known about the effects of chemical by-products of chlorine, we must depend on the EPA to ensure our safety. If newer research confirms the reports of increased birth defects from showering, swimming (*see* Swimming), and drinking water with high levels of THMs, stricter standards and testing will need to be enforced. If you are concerned, consider drinking bottled water or have your water tested. THM levels have been shown to be higher in pool water during busy use, so try to swim when the pool is less crowded. Outdoor pools and indoor pools with high ceilings may have lower concentrations of THMs in the air and may be a safer option.

Chocolate

Chocolate is food made from cocoa (*see* Cocoa) beans. It can be unsweetened or sweetened. To sweeten chocolate, milk, sugar, and vanilla are added.

CONCERNS: The main concern over chocolate consumption during pregnancy is that it is known to contain caffeine (*see* Caffeine). Other concerns focus around the fact that chocolate has a lot of calories and fat and can contain varying amounts of other chemicals, including theobromine, a chemical similar to caffeine. The average chocolate bar (28 grams) contains about 30 milligrams of caffeine.

A recent study from Finland noted an association between chocolate consumption during pregnancy and having a "positively reactive," or happier, baby at six months of age. The babies whose mothers had consumed chocolate during pregnancy demonstrated more smiling and laughter.

THE BOTTOM LINE: Chocolate, in moderation, is safe during pregnancy. Chocolate may also improve both your and your baby's happiness.

Chorionic villous sampling

Chorionic villous sampling (CVS) is a test usually performed by a high-risk maternal fetal medicine specialist (MFM) in which a needle is placed either through the mother's abdomen and into the placenta or through the cervix into the placenta. A small amount of fetal placental cells are withdrawn to allow for examination of fetal chromosomes that may detect some birth defects. CVS is usually performed at 10–12 weeks gestation, which is its main advantage over amniocentesis (*see* Amniocentesis).

Since CVS is performed to detect chromosomal abnormalities and not for treatment of an abnormality, you should be thoroughly counseled prior to undergoing this procedure and you should have an idea about what you will do with the information you receive. Some families would want this information to prepare for the child's life while other families may consider terminating the pregnancy if the results were not normal.

CONCERNS: Since this is an invasive procedure, the main concern centers on the risks of complications from the CVS procedure, including possible miscarriage. CVS has been associated with a higher miscarriage rate when compared to amniocentesis. However, a recent study looking at over 9,000 CVS procedures at a single institution showed that the rates of fetal loss were comparable to those of amniocentesis and that this new data may be due to specialists' increasing proficiency with the procedure. In this study the rate of pregnancy loss was found to be 1.93 percent, and when factors such as maternal age and indication for the procedure were matched, the rates of loss were the same for both CVS and amniocentesis.

THE BOTTOM LINE: CVS is not without risks. However, if the benefits outweigh the risks, it may be warranted. Pregnancy loss rates may be lower with specialists who have a lot of experience with the procedure and may be similar to those of amniocentesis.

Chromium ⚠️

Chromium is a mineral involved in the regulation of blood sugar that is found in many foods, including peanut butter, spinach, whole-wheat bread, apples, and chicken. A more toxic form exists as fine dust particles, as a result of manufacturing steel and other processes.

CONCERNS: New research suggests that chromium supplements may cause damage to the body's cells. Chromium toxicity can cause skin problems and cancer. Chromium dust inhaled from the air can cause respiratory problems and lung cancer. Chronic exposure may lead to gastrointestinal and skin problems and may affect the immune system. However, not much is known about the effects of chromium during pregnancy. The Environmental Protection Agency is involved in monitoring for harmful levels of chromium in the air. It suggests that you can minimize your risk by avoiding cigarette smoke, minimizing your exposure to vehicle exhaust, and containing copy machine toner dust.

THE BOTTOM LINE: The recommended daily allowance of chromium is 50 micrograms. This amount is easy to get in your diet, and a supplement appears to be unnecessary. Try to avoid exercise in areas with many cars and exhaust fumes.

Cipro®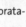

Cipro® is the brand name for the antibiotic ciprofloxacin (*see* Antibiotics, oral; Ciprofloxacin).

Ciprofloxacin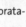

Ciprofloxacin is a quinolone antibiotic and is found in the brand Cipro® (*see* Antibiotics, oral).

CONCERNS: Ciprofloxacin has been assigned a risk factor category of C (*see* Appendix 1).

THE BOTTOM LINE: Ciprofloxacin is safe in pregnancy.

Claritin®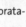

Claritin® is a brand name of loratadine (*see* Allergy medications; Loratadine).

Clavulanate potassium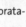

Clavulanate potassium is one of the antibiotics in the brand name antibiotic Augmentin® (*see* Augmentin; Antibiotics, oral).

CONCERNS: Clavulanate potassium has been assigned a risk factor category of B (*see* Appendix 1).

THE BOTTOM LINE: Clavulanate potassium is safe to take during pregnancy.

Cleaning products *See* Household cleaners.

Cleocin®

Cleocin® is the brand name for the antibiotic clindamycin (*see* Clindamycin; Antibiotics, topical).

Clindamycin ✓

Clindamycin is an antibiotic found in the brand name Cleocin® (*see* Antibiotics, topical).

CONCERNS: Data do not support an association between clindamycin use and birth defects. Clindamycin has been assigned a risk factor category of B (*see* Appendix 1).

THE BOTTOM LINE: Clindamycin is safe for use in pregnancy.

Cocaine ⃠

Cocaine is a drug that is made from coca leaves. It is a stimulant that is used medically as a local anesthetic and is also used as a drug of abuse (*see* Drugs of abuse). In powdered form, it can be inhaled, absorbed through the mucous membranes of the nose or gums, smoked, or injected directly into the bloodstream.

CONCERNS: Cocaine use has been clearly associated with pregnancy complications. These include miscarriage, preterm labor, preterm birth, hypertension, and placental abruption (premature separation of the placenta from the uterine wall). Cocaine use has been associated with fetal strokes, which can cause irreversible brain damage in the baby. Some studies have shown an increased risk of birth defects in children whose mothers used cocaine during their pregnancy, but these studies are not conclusive. Babies born to mothers who have used cocaine during their pregnancy are at increased risk for being irritable and are at risk for sudden infant death syndrome (SIDS). Some studies suggest that cocaine exposure during pregnancy is associated with lower IQ scores and learning and behavioral difficulties.

THE BOTTOM LINE: Cocaine should be avoided during pregnancy.

Cocoa ✓

Cocoa is made from dried and powdered cocoa beans. It can be sold plain or mixed with other ingredients, as in chocolate (*see* Chocolate).

CONCERNS: Cocoa contains caffeine (*see* Caffeine), which should be limited to 300 milligrams (mg) or less per day during pregnancy. The amounts of caffeine in prepared cocoa mix can vary:

- Chocolate powder mix (three heaping teaspoons) has 8 mg caffeine.
- One envelope of hot cocoa mix has 5 mg caffeine.

THE BOTTOM LINE: Moderate amounts of cocoa ingestion are safe in pregnancy.

Cod liver oil

Cod liver oil is oil that is extracted from the codfish. Cod liver oil can be purchased in health food stores in a capsule form. This oil can also be consumed by eating fish (see Fish). Cod liver oil contains elongated omega-3 fatty acids, preformed Vitamin A (see Vitamin A), Vitamin D (see Vitamin D) and Vitamin K (see Vitamin K).

CONCERNS: Since cod liver oil is rich in preformed Vitamin A, its use in pregnancy is of concern. Vitamin A can be found in two forms: preformed or retinoid, which originates from animal tissue and can be obtained through meat and dairy foods and from vitamin supplements and supplemented foods, and retinol, which is made in the body from beta-carotene (see Beta-carotene) and can be obtained from fruits, vegetables, and vitamin supplements. Preformed Vitamin A is considered to be a teratogen (causing birth defects) in high doses. However, the amount needed to cause birth defects is controversial. One study has shown that women who took 10,000 international units (3,000 RE) per day during pregnancy were five times more likely to have a child with a birth defect. The Teratology Society has estimated that taking greater than 25,000 international units (7,500 RE) per day of preformed Vitamin A in pregnancy would cause one in fifty-seven infants to have a birth defect. The U.S. Food and Drug Administration has set the recommended daily allowance of preformed Vitamin A to be 8,000 international units (2,400 RE) per day during pregnancy.

Cod is a fish that is low in methylmercury (see Methylmercury). Cod liver oil supplements do not appear to increase your risk of mercury toxicity.

Several studies noted an association between taking cod liver oil supplements during pregnancy and healthier babies. Specifically, these infants had a decreased risk of developing diabetes and had higher mental functioning at the age of four.

The consumption of certain oils can be used as a laxative (*see* Laxatives) and cause diarrhea, dehydration, preterm contractions, and preterm labor. If you experience diarrhea from cod liver oil, it is probably wise to decrease the amount that you are taking.

THE BOTTOM LINE: Cod liver oil in small amounts appears to be safe and may even be beneficial during pregnancy.

Codeine

Codeine is a narcotic drug used as a cough suppressant (*see* Cough and cold suppressants) and as a pain reliever (*see* Pain relievers). It is also commonly combined with Tylenol® (*see* Acetaminophen).

CONCERNS: Codeine has been assigned a risk factor category of C throughout pregnancy and a risk factor of D if used for prolonged periods or close to term (*see* Appendix 1). Several studies have demonstrated an association between codeine use and birth defects. However, these studies need to be confirmed, and many have not been found to be statistically significant. Narcotic withdrawal in the infant has been seen with mothers who took codeine for long periods of time and/or shortly before giving birth.

THE BOTTOM LINE: It is safe to take codeine as prescribed during pregnancy, but use caution if needed for long periods of time or close to delivery.

Coenzyme Q10

Also known as ubiquinone or CoQ10, coenzyme Q10 is a naturally occurring compound that is found in the mitochondria (energy-producing components) of all cells. It can also be found in oily fish (*see* Fish), organ meats, and whole grains, or a supplement can be taken in the form of capsules, sprays, or tablets. Most people consume adequate amounts from their diets, but some people use supplements in the belief that supplementation may boost energy, enhance the immune system, and act as an antioxidant. Some studies have shown this supplement to be of benefit in congestive heart failure, hypertension, heart attack, and breast cancer.

CONCERNS: One study saw an increase in CoQ10 levels with each trimester of pregnancy. The study also noted a correlation between low levels and miscarriage and high levels with contractions. Low levels have also been associated with preeclampsia (hypertension, protein in the urine, and swelling).

Since coenzyme Q10 is categorized as a food supplement, it is not regulated by the U.S. Food and Drug Administration. Thus, there is no guarantee of the strength, purity, or safety of this product. You should inform your health care provider if you are taking any nutritional supplements. It is unknown whether this supplement is safe in pregnancy.

THE BOTTOM LINE: There are no data to document CoQ10's safety for use during pregnancy. Use with caution until more studies are available.

Coffee

Coffee is a beverage made from ground, roasted coffee beans. It can be served hot or iced. It can be flavored with sugar, milk, cream, and other ingredients.

CONCERNS: Coffee contains caffeine (*see* Caffeine), unless it is decaffeinated. One study found an association between drinking more than eight cups of coffee per day and an increased risk of stillbirth. However, most scientists have found that consuming 300 milligrams (mg) or less of caffeine per day appears to be safe. Because the amount of caffeine varies in each cup of coffee, it is difficult to estimate how much you are consuming. On average, the amount can range from 57 to 350 mg caffeine per 8-ounce serving of coffee. Espresso or cappuccino has about 100 mg caffeine per 1.5- to 2-ounce serving.

THE BOTTOM LINE: One cup of caffeinated coffee per day appears to be safe. Decaffeinated coffee is safe during pregnancy.

Cola

Cola is a sweet carbonated beverage containing cola nut (*see* Cola nut) extract and other flavorings.

CONCERNS: Unless the label says the beverage is decaffeinated, colas contain caffeine (*see* Caffeine). There are approximately 30 to 100 milligrams (mg) caffeine per 12 ounces of cola. "High-energy" colas can contain as much as 100 mg caffeine.

Another consideration is the artificial sweeteners (*see* Artificial sweeteners) used in diet colas. Moderate amounts of Equal® or NutraSweet® (*see* Aspartame) ingestion have not been associated with pregnancy complications. Splenda® (*see* Sucralose) has not been associated with any pregnancy complications. Saccharin (*see* Saccharin) has been associated with birth defects in laboratory animals.

Keep in mind that colas with sugar contain a lot of "empty" calories. You might be better off consuming calories that have more nutritional value during pregnancy.

THE BOTTOM LINE: Consumption of 300 mg caffeine per day during pregnancy appears to be safe. Consumption of one diet drink containing aspartame or sucralose per day appears to be safe. Avoid diet drinks that contain saccharin.

Cola nut

The cola nut is the fruit of the cola tree. Some people chew on this nut, claiming it gives them energy and acts like an aphrodisiac. Cola nut extract is used for flavoring cola (*see* Cola).

CONCERNS: The extract of the cola nut contains caffeine (*see* Caffeine) and theobromine, a compound that is similar to caffeine. The amount of caffeine varies with the variety of nut and whether the nut is fresh or dried. The percent of caffeine can range from 1 to 5 percent. One report showed that ingesting 150 grains or 9.8 grams of cola nut caused cardiac problems.

THE BOTTOM LINE: Consuming less than 300 milligrams caffeine per day is safe in pregnancy.

Colace®

Colace® is a brand name for docusate (*see* Docusate; Laxatives).

Cold cuts *See* Cured meat; Deli meats, cooked and uncooked. ⚠

Cold-Eeze® ⚠

Cold-Eeze® is a cold remedy taken orally that contains 4.34 mg of zinc (*see* Zinc). Zinc is thought to affect the immune system and act as an antioxidant. Cold-Eeze® claims to shorten the common cold by 3–4 days.

CONCERNS: Concerns over Cold-Eeze® center on the affects of extra zinc in your diet during pregnancy. If you take the product as directed, you will ingest more than the Recommended Daily Allowance (RDA) of zinc for pregnancy. Despite this concern over consuming more than the RDA of zinc per day, zinc is relatively nontoxic and has no known association with genetic abnormalities. Excess zinc may affect the level of maternal pancreatic enzymes, lipoproteins, and the immune system.

The second concern is that this product is considered a food supplement and is not regulated by the U.S. Food and Drug Administration (FDA). Thus there is no guarantee of the strength, purity, or safety of this product. You should inform your health care provider if you are taking any nutritional supplements.

THE BOTTOM LINE: Although Cold-Eeze® is probably safe during pregnancy, there is little information about its use during pregnancy to support or discourage its use.

Colonics ⚠

Several different types of colonics are used to cleanse the intestines. Some people believe that our small bowel and large colon (intestines) need to be cleaned periodically to increase wellness and prevent disease.

CONCERNS: Some providers of colon hydrotherapy state that colonics are contraindicated in the first trimester, but they do not provide a reason for this. Other providers report that its use is safe in pregnancy, unless the pregnancy is high risk.

No scientific literature examining the effect of colonics during pregnancy could be found. Consequently, caution should be used. Some procedures may result in dehydration, which can sometimes trigger preterm contractions.

THE BOTTOM LINE: Although colonics are probably safe during pregnancy, very little is known about them and their effects during pregnancy. It is probably best to avoid them, especially if you are at risk for preterm labor.

Computers ✓

Computer screens are used to display the output of the computer to the user. They work in a similar fashion to the television, using a cathode ray tube (CRT) to transmit images. CRTs work by moving an electron beam back and forth across the back of the screen. Each time the beam makes a pass across the screen, it lights up phosphor dots on the inside of the glass tube, thereby illuminating the active portions of the screen. By drawing many such lines from the top to the bottom of the screen, the beam creates an entire screen of images. Plasma screens or flat screens use glass chambers filled with neon and xenon gas. When energized, the chambers emit UV light that energizes red, green, and blue phosphors on the back of the display glass producing visible light.

CONCERNS: Several concerns have been raised over the use of computer screens during pregnancy. These concerns include a possible association with birth defects, effects of radiation exposure, eye strain, back strain, and carpal tunnel syndrome.

A few reported cases of birth defects and miscarriages have been associated with computer use. An ongoing study by the National Institute for Occupational Safety and Health is examining this question. When the study is completed, more information will be available. According to specialists in radiation safety, computers emit midrange microwave radiation, not X rays (*see* X rays). This type of radiation is not a risk for birth defects or miscarriage.

The risks of eye strain, back strain, and carpal tunnel syndrome due to computer use exist even when you are not pregnant. However, you may be more susceptible to strains when pregnant due to your changing center of gravity and to increased levels of the hormone relaxin, which loosens ligaments and can make it easier to hurt yourself. Good advice for everyone is to take periodic breaks while working at the computer.

THE BOTTOM LINE: Although computer screens are probably safe during pregnancy, you can take a few precautions to minimize your risks. Sit as far back from the screen as you can, use a comfortable chair, and stretch every 30 minutes or so.

Conjugated linoleic acid

Conjugated linoleic acid (CLA) is a form of the essential fatty acid linoleic acid. CLA is naturally found in dairy products, beef, poultry, eggs, and corn oil. Some people take supplements to limit food allergies, prevent atherosclerosis, and improve glucose tolerance.

CONCERNS: Many studies have examined CLA supplementation in pregnant and lactating farm animals. Human studies have demonstrated that CLA levels rise throughout pregnancy. One study demonstrated that women with preeclampsia (hypertension, protein in the urine, and swelling) had higher levels of CLA compared to controls.

Since conjugated linoleic acid is categorized as a food supplement, it is not regulated by the U.S. Food and Drug Administration. Thus, there is no guarantee of the strength, purity, or safety of this product. You should inform your health care provider if you are taking any nutritional supplements.

THE BOTTOM LINE: There are no clear data on the safety of CLA supplementation during pregnancy. Further, it is easy to get enough CLA from foods. Until more is known, supplementation is not necessary.

Contact lenses

An alternative to glasses, contact lenses are plastic or polymer lenses placed directly over the cornea of the eye.

CONCERNS: Some people believe that your immune system is weaker during pregnancy, and that could increase your risk of developing an eye infection. However, there are no clear data indicating that the immune response is either suppressed or increased during pregnancy. As when not pregnant, take the time to carefully clean and maintain your contact lenses.

A more realistic concern is related to the changes in your eyes during pregnancy. Some pregnant women experience increased dryness and swelling that can make wearing contacts uncomfortable.

THE BOTTOM LINE: Contact lenses are safe in pregnancy. If problems do arise, contact your OB/GYN or eye doctor for evaluation. You may be advised to avoid your contacts until after you deliver or use rewetting drops more frequently.

Cookie dough ⚠

Cookie dough is made from eggs (*see* Eggs), butter, sugar, flour, and other flavorings.

CONCERNS: Because cookie dough often contains raw eggs, there is a possibility that it could contain a bacterium called *Salmonella* (*see* Salmonella). *Salmonella* can cause diarrhea, fever, and abdominal pain. It is most dangerous in people who have a weakened immune system. Women who are pregnant do not appear to be at an increased risk of getting *Salmonella*. However, one type of this bacterium can cross the placenta and cause miscarriage, stillbirth, and preterm labor. Cooking any food to 165°F/74°C will destroy *Salmonella* instantly.

THE BOTTOM LINE: Commercial cookie dough products, including cookie dough ice cream, are made with pasteurized eggs and are not a problem. When cooking with raw eggs, avoid tasting raw cookie dough and clean up properly to avoid contamination of utensils and working surfaces.

Cough and cold suppressants ⚠

Cough and cold suppressants are generally sold over the counter to reduce the symptoms associated with upper respiratory tract infections caused by viruses. Often they contain several medicines in varying combinations, including expectorants (*see* Expectorants), antitussives (*see* Antitussives), antihistamines (*see* Antihistamines), decongestants (*see* Decongestants), and analgesics (*see* Pain relievers). Preparations include Advil® Cold & Sinus, Comtrex®, Contac®, Nyquil®, Robitussin®, Theraflu®, and various generic names. Knowing the individual ingredients will help you to determine which cold medicines are safe and which should be avoided.

CONCERNS: Cough and cold suppressants contain many types of ingredients.

- *Expectorants* break up chest secretions and have not been clearly associated with birth defects or pregnancy complications. Guaifenesin (*see* Guaifenesin) is the main ingredient in most over-the-counter expectorants. Brands include Antituss® and Robitussin®.

- *Antitussives* are used to suppress coughs and are also considered safe in pregnancy. Dextromethorphan (*see* Dextromethorphan) is the main ingredient in most over-the-counter antitussives while codeine (*see* Codeine) and hydrocodone can be found in many prescription drugs. Brand names include Benylin®, Cough-X®, and Robitussin®.

- *Antihistamines* decrease itching and are generally assigned a risk factor category of B or C (*see* Appendix 1). They have not been clearly associated with birth defects or pregnancy complications. Antihistamines include Allegra® (*see* Fexofenadine), Claritin® (*see* Loratadine), and Zyrtec® (*see* Cetrizine).

- *Decongestants* act to constrict blood vessels to decrease swelling and mucus production and have not been clearly associated with birth defects or pregnancy complications. However, there is a theoretical concern that their vasoconstrictive (ability to constrict blood vessels) properties could cause some complications and so it is advised that they be used sparingly, especially in the third trimester. Decongestant sprays may be safer than oral dosing due to decreased amounts of absorbed drug. A common decongestant is pseudoephedrine (*see* Pseudoephedrine), which can be found in Chlor-trimeton®, Dimetapp®, Sudafed®, and Triaminic®.

- *Analgesics* act to treat aches and pains, and most are not associated with birth defects. Tylenol® (*see* Acetaminophen) is the pain reliever of choice in pregnancy. Avoid Bayer® (*see* Aspirin), Advil®, Motrin®, and Nuprin® (*see* Ibuprofen); and Aleve® (*see* Naproxen), especially in the third trimester.

- *Alcohol* (*see* Alcoholic beverages) can be found in some over-the-counter cold remedies, including liquid Nyquil. Most health care providers recommend that you avoid consumption of alcohol during pregnancy.

THE BOTTOM LINE: Most cough and cold suppressants are considered safe in pregnancy. Consult with your health care provider regarding any specific medications. It is best to limit medication use by choosing drugs that treat specific symptoms and using them only when needed.

Creatine monohydrate

Creatine can be found in the body as creatine kinase and creatine phosphate, which are enzymes that convert ATP (adenosine triphosphate) to energy and ADP (adenosine diphosphate) back to ATP respectively. ADP and ATP are compounds that are responsible for the transfer of energy in the body. Creatine is taken into the body by eating meat and fish. Some athletes feel that taking extra creatine in the form of creatine monohydrate can promote physical performance and stamina. It can be purchased in powder form.

CONCERNS: Since creatine monohydrate is categorized as a food supplement, it is not regulated by the U.S. Food and Drug Administration. Thus, there is no guarantee of the strength, purity, or safety of this product. It is a good idea to inform your health care provider if you are taking any nutritional supplements.

THE BOTTOM LINE: Not enough is known about creatine supplementation during pregnancy. Since there is no compelling reason to use this supplement during pregnancy, it is probably best to avoid it.

Cured meat

Cured meats are preserved through smoking, pickling, salting, or with nitrates and nitrites. Commonly cured meats include smoked ham, salami, corned beef, prosciutto, hot dogs (*see* Hot dogs), and bacon.

CONCERNS: Eating cured meats may be the number one way to contract the parasite *Toxoplasmosis gondii* (*see* Toxoplasmosis). Researchers have found that eating undercooked or cured meat accounts for 30 to 60 percent of *Toxoplasmosis* infections. *Toxoplasmosis* can cause fetal death, preterm labor, and some kinds of birth defects. However, keep in mind that *Toxoplasmosis* is a common childhood infection. Many people are immune to it, and a quick blood test from your health care provider will reveal whether you are immune.

Undercooked meat can also be contaminated with *Campylobacter*. *Campylobacter jejuni* bacteria (*see Campylobacter*; Bacteria) are responsible for a large number of food-poisoning and gastroenteritis cases. The most common food sources of these bacteria are undercooked meat and poultry, raw shellfish (*see* Shellfish), and unpasteurized milk and juice (*see* Unpasteurized juice). The bacteria can spread from person to person via inadequate hand washing.

Listeria monocytogenes (*see Listeria*) is a bacterium that can cause preterm labor and stillbirth during pregnancy. Pregnant women are 20 times more likely to get listeriosis than other healthy adults.

Listeria can contaminate cured meats despite proper storage and refrigeration. The risk of contamination can be decreased, but not prevented, by keeping your refrigerator at 40°F/4.5°C or below; keeping your refrigerator clean; avoiding cross-contamination from countertops, cutting boards (*see* Cutting boards), and utensils; and not leaving foods unrefrigerated for more than two hours.

Finally, meat cured with nitrates and nitrites (*see* Nitrates and nitrites), such as bacon and hot dogs, have been associated with low birth weights and methemoglobinemia (a blood disorder resulting in low oxygen) in laboratory animals.

THE BOTTOM LINE: The FDA recommends that all ready-to-eat meats be cooked until steaming to avoid several foodborne illnesses during pregnancy. It seems reasonable to avoid diets high in nitrate-cured meats while pregnant.

Cutting boards

Cutting boards are generally made of wood or plastic and are used for cutting meats and vegetables.

CONCERNS: Bacteria (*see* Bacteria) and parasites, including *Campylobacter* (*see* Campylobacter), *Salmonella* (*see* Salmonella), and *Toxoplasmosis gondii* (*see* Toxoplasmosis) can accumulate in the knife cuts in the boards. The bacteria can then contaminate other foods when the cutting board is used. Recent studies by the U.S. Food and Drug Administration (FDA) found that microorganisms became trapped in wood surfaces and were difficult to dislodge by rinsing; microorganisms were more easily washed off plastic surfaces. Based on these studies, the FDA released several recommendations for using cutting boards:

- Wash all cutting boards with hot, soapy water using a brush and allow to air dry or wipe dry with a clean paper towel. Wash nonporous acrylic, plastic, glass, and solid wood boards in an automatic dishwasher.

- Sanitize both wood and plastic cutting boards with diluted chlorine bleach or a vinegar solution. (Use 1 teaspoon liquid chlorine bleach to 4 cups water; use 1 cup vinegar to 5 cups water.) Flood the surface with a sanitizing solution and allow it to stand for several minutes, then rinse and air dry or pat dry with paper towels.

- Discard excessively worn cutting boards.

- Use a separate cutting board and knives for raw foods that require cooking. For example, use one for meat, poultry, or fish, and another for cooked or ready-to-eat foods such as salad, vegetables, and breads.

THE BOTTOM LINE: The use of properly cleaned cutting boards is safe in pregnancy.

Datril®

Datril® is a brand name for acetaminophen (*see* Acetaminophen).

Decongestants

Decongestants are found in many cold medicines and help to reduce nasal congestion (*see* Cough and cold suppressants). Pseudoephedrine (*see* Pseudoephedrine) is a common decongestant.

CONCERNS: Most decongestants are classified as risk factor category C (*see* Appendix 1).

THE BOTTOM LINE: Decongestants appear to be safe in pregnancy. Discuss individual decongestants with your health care provider.

DEET

DEET, or diethyltoluamide, is the active ingredient in many bug sprays and insect repellents (*see* Insect repellents.)

CONCERNS: Concern over the use of DEET increased after several reports of seizures in young children exposed to it. DEET is also known to be absorbed through the skin and can cross the placenta in animal studies. There is limited information about DEET use during pregnancy. However, in one known case, a child born to a woman who used DEET throughout her pregnancy had birth defects. Overall, DEET is considered to be safe for use during pregnancy and should be used, as the risks of DEET use appear to be less than those of West Nile virus, which is transmitted by infected mosquitoes.

DEET preparations come in varying concentrations, generally ranging from 5 to 30 percent, although higher concentrations are available. The recommendations for young children are to use the lowest concentration available and apply to clothes and not directly to skin. However, keep in mind that the lower concentrations are active for shorter periods of time and may need to be reapplied after a couple of hours. Reapplication may be necessary after prolonged time spent outside or after swimming.

The Centers for Disease Control and Prevention has the following recommendations for using insect repellents:

- Use enough repellent to cover exposed skin or clothing. Don't apply repellent to skin that is under clothing. Heavy application is not necessary to achieve protection.
- Do not apply repellent to cuts, wounds, or irritated skin. After returning indoors, wash treated skin with soap and water.
- Do not spray aerosol or pump products in enclosed areas.
- Do not spray aerosol or pump products directly on your face. Spray your hands and then rub them carefully over the face, avoiding eyes and mouth.

THE BOTTOM LINE: DEET is not contraindicated in pregnancy. Use as instructed, try to limit exposure, and wash hands carefully after application.

Dehumidifiers

Dehumidifiers are machines that remove moisture from the air. They are often used in environments that contain a lot of water or humidity, such as basements.

CONCERNS: As with air conditioners and humidifiers (*see* Air conditioners; Humidifiers), there has been some publicity about the association of Legionnaire's disease outbreaks with dehumidifiers. Legionnaire's disease is caused by a bacterium called *legionellae*, which lives in warm-water environments like those found in air conditioners, plumbing systems, and humidifiers. It is estimated that 8,000 to 10,000 people contract Legionnaire's disease every year. However, it is often difficult to diagnose the disease accurately because symptoms can vary from person to person. Unless a doctor specifically suspects Legionnaire's, the appropriate tests are often not performed. The disease is most dangerous to those who have a weakened immune system due to cancer therapy, smoking, or organ transplant. Pregnancy does not appear to be an increased risk factor for getting this disease. While the U.S. Department of Labor's Occupational Safety and Health Administration has standards in place for work-related systems, it is unclear how many cases of Legionnaire's disease are acquired in private homes and what the optimal methods of prevention are. Proper maintenance of all plumbing systems, air-conditioning systems, and humidifiers should minimize your risk of contracting this disease.

Dehumidifiers are also great places for mold to grow. Some people are allergic to mold, so your dehumidifier should be properly cleaned and maintained. Follow the manufacturer's suggestions for proper maintenance.

THE BOTTOM LINE: A well-maintained dehumidifier is safe in pregnancy and may be beneficial for reducing humidity.

Deli meats, cooked and uncooked ⚠

Deli meats refer to ready-to-eat meats sold in packages and at deli counters. These include cured meats (*see* Cured meat) like smoked ham, prosciutto, and salami, hot dogs (*see* Hot dogs), roasted and smoked turkey, and roast beef.

CONCERNS: A study in 2001 by the Food Safety and Inspection Service of the United States Department of Agriculture (FSIS/USDA) determined that many pregnant women were either not aware of the dangers of certain foods or did not handle these foods properly in the home. It is important to know that you are at risk for several food-borne illnesses that can be contracted through deli meats during pregnancy.

Cured meats can contain parasites such as *Toxoplasmosis* (*see Toxoplasmosis*) and bacteria such as *Listeria* (*see Listeria*) and *Campylobacter* (*see Campylobacter*), all of which can cause preterm labor, miscarriage, and stillbirth. Researchers have found that eating undercooked or cured meat accounts for 30 to 60 percent of *Toxoplasmosis* infections. Pregnant women are 20 times more likely to get *Listeria* than other healthy adults.

Deli meats are also susceptible to *Listeria* from contamination by meat slicers, cutting boards, knives, and refrigerators. *Listeria* can contaminate these foods despite proper storage and refrigeration. The risk of contamination can be decreased, but not prevented, by keeping your refrigerator at 40°F/4.5°C or below; keeping your refrigerator clean; avoiding cross-contamination from countertops, cutting boards (*see* Cutting boards), and utensils; and not leaving foods unrefrigerated for more than two hours. Deli meats should be well cooked prior to eating.

The USDA and the U.S. Food and Drug Administration recommend that pregnant women:

- Don't eat hot dogs or deli meats unless reheated and steaming hot.
- Don't eat refrigerated patés or meat spreads. Only canned paté (*see* Paté) and meat spreads that do not require refrigeration are safe.

THE BOTTOM LINE: Careful cooking prior to eating will eliminate any worry about eating deli meats during pregnancy. Do not eat deli meats unless they are reheated and steaming hot. Remember to clean up properly so you do not contaminate other foods with unwashed cutting boards (*see* Cutting boards) and knives.

Dentists

Approximately 42 percent of the population in the United States had at least one dental visit in 2000. Further, women are more likely to visit dentists than men.

CONCERNS: Concern over routine X rays (*see* X rays), anesthetic gases (*see* Anesthetic gases, use of), and dental treatments has led to fears about going to the dentist during pregnancy. However, most dental care is perfectly safe during pregnancy. Despite the low levels of radiation during dental X rays, most dentists avoid routine X rays during pregnancy. However, if there is a specific problem and X rays are recommended, they are considered to be safe with abdominal shielding. Local anesthesia (*see* Anesthetic, local) without epinephrine is also considered to be safe during pregnancy. It is a good idea to avoid elective dental work during pregnancy to reduce your exposure to anesthetic gases and radiation.

Dental work during the first trimester is probably fine. However, most dentists recommend waiting until the second trimester (after 12 weeks) to limit concern over possible teratogenic (cause of birth defects) effects of anesthetics or treatments. Dental work in the third trimester is often difficult secondary to discomfort in lying in the dental chair.

Periodontal disease has been associated with preterm labor, and its prevention is another reason to visit the dentist during pregnancy. Oral infections should be treated to prevent spread to the rest of the body and potential adverse fetal effects.

Finally, there has been some concern over silver fillings, which can contain as much as 52 percent mercury (*see* Mercury). However, the American Dental Association has researched this topic and has failed to detect any significant problems related to the mercury in the fillings.

THE BOTTOM LINE: It is safe and healthy to visit your dentist for regular dental care or as needed.

Desoxyn®

Desoxyn® is a brand name of amphetamine (*see* Amphetamines).

Dexadrine®

Dexadrine® is a brand name of amphetamine (*see* Amphetamines).

Dextromethorphan

Dextromethorphan is the most commonly used antitussive (*see* Antitussives; Cough and cold suppressants) in over-the-counter cough medicines. It is used to suppress coughs. Dextromethorphan is found in many cough and cold suppressants, including Benylyn®, Cough-X®, and Robitussin®.

CONCERNS: The risk factor category assigned to dextromethorphan is C (*see* Appendix 1).

THE BOTTOM LINE: Dextromethorphan is considered to be safe during pregnancy.

DHEA

DHEA (dehydroepiandrosterone) is a steroid hormone precursor. Due to an association of decreased levels of DHEA with cancer, aging, and cardiovascular disease, some people use this as a supplement for improved health. It is thought to enhance energy, sex drive, and sports performance. It can be purchased in capsule form.

CONCERNS: Clinical studies using DHEA to treat a variety of conditions have had inconsistent results. One author noted a decline in DHEA following pregnancy and postulated that these lower levels may be responsible for preterm labor following pregnancies that are close together. However, DHEA has also been found to increase androgen levels in women and may enhance the progression of estrogen- and testosterone-sensitive cancers.

Since DHEA is categorized as a food supplement, it is not regulated by the FDA. Thus, there is no guarantee of the strength, purity, or safety of this product. You should inform your health care provider if you are taking any nutritional supplements.

THE BOTTOM LINE: DHEA is considered to be contraindicated during pregnancy and should be avoided.

Diethyltoluamide *See* DEET; Insect repellents; Insecticides.

Dieting

Dieting generally refers to the restriction of calories or food groups with the goal of losing weight.

CONCERNS: Because you need extra calories and a variety of nutrients when you are pregnant, calorie-restrictive dieting is not generally advised. On average, you require an additional 300 calories per day. It is recommended that you gain 25 to 35 pounds during pregnancy, depending on your prepregnancy weight. Poor weight gain has been associated with intrauterine growth restriction (low birth weight) and preterm delivery.

One study showed that women who dieted early in their pregnancy had twice the risk of having a baby with a neural tube defect, probably due to a lower intake of vitamins and nutrients.

THE BOTTOM LINE: Dieting is not recommended during pregnancy and may be associated with an increased risk of birth defects. A healthy diet with extra protein, calcium, fruits, and vegetables is recommended by most health care providers.

Diflucan®

Diflucan® is the brand name for fluconazole (*see* Fluconazole; Antifungal medications, oral and topical).

Diving *See* Scuba diving.

Docusate

Docusate is a stool softener used in the treatment of constipation (*see* Laxatives). A common brand name of docusate is Colace®.

CONCERNS: The risk factor category assigned to docusate is C (*see* Appendix 1). Constipation is a common complaint for many women during pregnancy, perhaps because of changes in diet and exercise levels. Iron and calcium supplements have also been blamed for causing constipation. Increases in the hormone progesterone during pregnancy may also play a role in slowing down your intestinal tract. Most gastroenterologists suggest that increasing your fiber intake is the best way to treat constipation.

THE BOTTOM LINE: Docusate is considered to be safe in pregnancy.

Dogs

Based on a 2001–2002 national pet owners survey, there were an estimated 68 million dogs living as pets in the United States. Forty percent of households had at least one dog as a pet.

CONCERNS: One concern about dogs centers around dog bites. Dog bites often require medical care and can result in hospitalization and even death. Seventy-seven percent of biting dogs belonged to the victim's family or friend. These events are not related to pregnancy and occur at any time.

A second concern centers around the use of flea and tick medication (*see* Flea and tick medication). Women exposed to household insecticides (*see* Insecticides, home use) are 1.5 times more likely to have a child with a birth defect. The most common defects noted were neural tube defects, facial defects, and limb defects. The greatest risk appears to be with exposure during the first trimester and with prolonged exposure. A recent study showed an association between using flea/tick collars with pediatric brain tumors. This risk was highest for women who applied the flea collars themselves.

Finally, animal stool can be contaminated with the bacterium *Campylobacter jejuni* (*see* Campylobacter), a common cause of gastroenteritis. Wash hands carefully after picking up after your dog.

THE BOTTOM LINE: Dogs are safe in pregnancy. Avoid aggressive dogs. Avoid applying flea and tick collars and using insecticides while pregnant.

Douches

Douching is the process of cleaning the vagina using a variety of solutions, including water, vinegar, baking soda, and store-bought douches. It is estimated that 37 percent of American women douche on a regular basis.

CONCERNS: Despite the fact that a large number of women douche, most OB/GYNs consider this to be unnecessary and even harmful. Douching can change the normal acid-alkaline balance in the vagina and make you more at risk for developing infections like bacterial vaginitis (BV) (*see* Bacterial vaginitis). BV has been clearly associated with an increased risk of preterm labor. Douching may also increase your risk of pelvic inflammatory disease (PID) and ectopic pregnancy (pregnancy outside the uterus). Studies have also shown an association between douching during pregnancy and both preterm labor and low-birth-weight babies.

THE BOTTOM LINE: Douching should be avoided during pregnancy.

Drugs of abuse

 ⃠ ⚠

Drugs of abuse are substances that are used to alter one's mental state. Many are illegal; others are available by prescription, and "abuse" refers to their use without a physician's advice or approval. Common drugs of abuse include amphetamines (*see* Amphetamines), cocaine (*see* Cocaine), heroin, marijuana (*see* Marijuana), and alcohol (*see* Alcoholic beverages).

CONCERNS: Many of these drugs have been associated with pregnancy complications and behavioral problems in the children of mothers who abuse these drugs, but information regarding their safety is limited. While prescription drugs are rated and assigned an individual risk factor category by the U.S. Food and Drug Administration, many drugs of abuse do not have the same monitoring. Like food supplements, there is no guarantee as to the strength, purity, or effectiveness of these drugs. Further, these drugs are generally illegal in the United States.

Another factor that complicates determining their effects during pregnancy is that most people who use drugs of abuse also smoke tobacco, drink alcohol, and have poor nutrition and limited prenatal care. These additional factors make it difficult to tease out the effects of individual drugs.

- *Amphetamines* are a group of drugs that are used as a central nervous system stimulant. They are used for several medical conditions, such as narcolepsy (a sleep disorder) and attention deficit hyperactivity disorder (ADHD), and as an appetite suppressant. Women with substance abuse issues may abuse amphetamines. Infants born to women with recent amphetamine use show signs of agitation and can experience withdrawal symptoms. Some small studies have shown an increase in structural birth defects with amphetamine use. There does seem to be an increased risk of preterm labor, intrauterine growth restriction (low birth weight), and fetal cerebrovascular events (events relating to the blood vessels of the brain, i.e., strokes). The risk factor category for this drug is C (*see* Appendix 1).

- *Ecstasy* is an amphetamine, or stimulant. There is limited information on its use during pregnancy. One report from the United Kingdom indicated that there was an increased risk of limb defects associated with Ecstasy use during the first trimester. A small study found a possible increase in heart defects.

- *Cocaine* is a stimulant that has been associated with preterm labor, preterm birth, hypertension, and placental abruption. Cocaine use is also associated with low-birth-weight babies, as they do not get the oxygen and nutrients that they need. After birth, some babies that are exposed to cocaine are irritable and go through a withdrawal period and require special care in the neonatal intensive care unit (NICU). There is some evidence that cocaine use may be associated with structural birth defects, but this has not been clearly proven.

- *Heroin* is a narcotic. Heroin use during pregnancy has been associated with intrauterine growth restriction (low birth weight), preterm delivery, and stillbirth. Its use during pregnancy has also been associated with behavioral abnormalities later in childhood. Heroin has not been associated with structural birth defects. Babies are often born addicted to this drug and may require special care in a NICU.

- *Marijuana* is a plant that is dried and smoked. Smoking marijuana prior to pregnancy has been associated with decreased male and female fertility. Several studies have associated marijuana use during pregnancy with low-birth-weight babies and neurological delays. Smaller babies are more prone to develop health problems in childhood and adulthood. However, despite these associations, studies have been mixed. One large retrospective study that was able to show an association between low birth weight and marijuana use found that when patients who also used tobacco were eliminated from the study results, an association was no longer seen. Occasional use of marijuana has not been associated with structural birth defects.

- *Alcohol* is a known teratogen (cause of birth defects). Regular alcohol consumption and binge drinking during pregnancy have been associated with fetal alcohol syndrome (FAS). Currently there is no known safe amount of alcohol during pregnancy, and pregnant women are advised not to consume any alcohol during pregnancy.

THE BOTTOM LINE: Most drugs of abuse appear to have some effect on the fetus. Information regarding their safety is limited. Since this is an avoidable risk, avoid the substances while pregnant. If you feel that you need help in doing this, please seek out help from your health care provider.

Dry cleaning

Dry cleaning is a process of cleaning clothes using little water. Commonly used chemicals include perchloroethylene, tetrachloroethylene, and benzene (*see* Benzene).

CONCERNS: Many of the chemicals used in dry cleaning are volatile organic compounds (VOCs). The health effects of VOCs can vary greatly, ranging from highly toxic to no known health effects. The health effects of VOCs will depend on the nature of the volatile organic compound, the level of exposure, and length of exposure.

According to the Tenth Report on Carcinogens by the Department of Health and Human Services, benzene is known to be a human carcinogen, and perchloroethylene is reasonably anticipated to be a carcinogen. People at the highest risk of long-term exposure to these VOCs are industrial workers who handle the compounds in the workplace, cigarette smokers, and people who spend much time exposed to emissions from heavy motor vehicle traffic.

THE BOTTOM LINE: Dry cleaning uses many dangerous chemicals. However, the risks appear to be related to length of time and amount of exposure. Fortunately, the amount of chemicals remaining on your clothes after dry cleaning appears to be negligible. Airing out your clothes prior to wearing them and limiting the number of times that you dry-clean a garment will help minimize your exposure. Pregnant women who work around these chemicals should use caution, as organic solvents have been associated with miscarriage and birth defects.

E. coli **infection** ⚠️

Escherichia coli is a bacterium (*see* Bacteria). Most strains are harmless, but some can cause food-borne illness. Infection with certain strains of *E. coli* is characterized by bloody diarrhea and can occasionally cause kidney failure due to the production of a toxin. *E. coli* can be acquired through contaminated foods such as unpasteurized juices, ground beef, raw sprouts (*see* Sprouts, raw), and swimming (*see* Swimming) in or drinking contaminated water.

CONCERNS: In some rare cases of preterm labor, *E. coli* has been isolated from the amniotic fluid. You are not more likely to get an infection with *E. coli* during pregnancy compared to other healthy adults.

THE BOTTOM LINE: Infection with *E. coli* can be dangerous, but is not more likely during pregnancy. Ground beef should be cooked until the thickest part reads 160°F/71°C with a meat thermometer. Clean work surfaces and utensils carefully to avoid cross-contamination while preparing food. Avoid drinking unpasteurized juices and eating raw sprouts during pregnancy. Wash raw vegetables prior to eating them.

Echinacea ⚠️

Echinacea is an herb used as a medication. It is obtained from the plant *Echinacea*, which comes in several varieties. Echinacea is used to stimulate the immune system during colds and upper respiratory infections. Echinacea can be taken as a capsule, extract, tincture, or as a tea (*see* Herb tea).

CONCERNS: A few studies have looked at echinacea use during pregnancy. So far, its use has not been associated with any birth defects, but these studies are retrospective, and there is little information documenting echinacea's safety. Tinctures of echinacea contain alcohol (*see* Alcoholic beverages), which should be avoided during pregnancy.

Echinacea is characterized as a dietary supplement, and as such it is not regulated by the U.S. Food and Drug Administration (FDA). Thus, there is no guarantee of the strength, purity, or safety of this product. You should inform your health care provider if you are taking any nutritional supplements. As its use is widespread, the FDA has examined the scientific literature on echinacea and has assigned it a risk factor category of C (*see* Appendix 1).

THE BOTTOM LINE: In the limited information available on the use of echinacea during pregnancy, no association with birth defects or problems could be found.

Effexor® ⚠

Effexor® is a brand name for venlafaxine (*see* Psychiatric medications).

Eggnog ⚠

Eggnog is a seasonal drink made from milk or cream, eggs (*see* Eggs), sugar, nutmeg, and usually alcohol (*see* Alcoholic beverages) of some kind.

CONCERNS: There are two concerns about eggnog: the use of raw eggs and the use of alcohol. Raw eggs may contain the bacterium *Salmonella* (*see* Salmonella), which can cause diarrhea, fever, and abdominal pain. It is most dangerous in people who have a weakened immune system. Women who are pregnant do not appear to be at an increased risk of getting *Salmonella*. However, one type of this bacterium can cross the placenta and cause miscarriage, stillbirth, and preterm labor.

Fetal alcohol syndrome (FAS) is a syndrome that includes intrauterine growth restriction (low birth weight) and brain abnormalities and is clearly associated with frequent alcohol consumption or binge drinking.

Many health care providers recommend that no alcohol be consumed during pregnancy because it is not clearly known how much alcohol is safe in pregnancy.

THE BOTTOM LINE: Avoid eggnog made with raw eggs or with alcohol. Commercially available products use pasteurized egg products and are safe.

Eggs

Eggs are eaten alone or as an ingredient in many homemade and commercially prepared foods. Eggs have a high moisture content, which can promote the growth of bacteria.

CONCERNS: The Centers for Disease Control and Prevention (CDC) estimates that 1 in 20,000 eggs is infected with *Salmonella enteritidis* (*see Salmonella*). This bacterium can be transmitted by infected hens and can affect any egg, including those with clean and intact shells. Although infection with *Salmonella* has not been associated with birth defects, it has been shown to cause miscarriage, preterm labor, and stillbirth.

In order to avoid eating contaminated eggs, the U.S. Food and Drug Administration (FDA) suggests the following guidelines:

- Wash hands, utensils, and countertops with warm, soapy water before and after coming into contact with raw eggs.
- Cook all eggs thoroughly until the yolks and whites are firm.
- Cook fried eggs two to three minutes per side or four minutes in a covered pan.
- Cook scrambled eggs until firm throughout.
- Cook hard-boiled eggs for seven minutes.
- Don't taste foods made with raw, unpasteurized eggs while cooking.
- Pregnant women should avoid eating raw cookie dough (*see* Cookie dough), homemade dressings (*see* Caesar salad; Homemade mayonnaise), homemade ice cream (*see* Homemade ice cream), meringue (*see* Meringue), and mousse (*see* Mousse).

- Commercially prepared products generally use pasteurized eggs and are safe. You can purchase pasteurized eggs, which are safe in pregnancy.

THE BOTTOM LINE: Avoid all raw and undercooked unpasteurized eggs and foods containing them during pregnancy. Commercially available products use pasteurized egg products and are safe. Store eggs properly below 40°F/4.5°C and use before their freshness date passes.

Elavil® ⊘

Elavil® is a brand name for amitriptyline (see Psychiatric medications).

Electric and magnetic fields ☑

All electric household appliances create an electric and magnetic field (EMF).

CONCERNS: It has been postulated that EMFs could cause cell damage and possibly cancer. However, no studies have been able to clearly demonstrate this association. EMFs have been associated with childhood acute lymphoblastic anemia (ALL). A 1998 study that looked at the effects of EMFs during pregnancy found no association between household appliance use and ALL.

THE BOTTOM LINE: EMFs have not been proven to be harmful during pregnancy.

Electric blankets ⚠ ∴

Electric blankets contain a connection to an electric source to create increased warmth.

CONCERNS: A recent study found an increased rate of miscarriage with use of electric blankets around the time of conception and during the first trimester. Although it is unclear why this is, two possibilities are the existence of electric and magnetic fields (EMFs) (see Electric and magnetic fields) and increased temperature.

It has been postulated that EMFs could cause cell damage and possibly cancer. However, no studies have been able to clearly demonstrate this association. EMFs have been associated with childhood acute lymphoblastic anemia (ALL). A 1998 study that looked at the effects of EMFs during pregnancy found no association between household appliance use, including electric blanket use, and ALL.

Electric blankets may increase maternal core body temperature, which has been associated with such fetal abnormalities as neural tube defects. Therefore, avoiding their use during the first trimester seems to be a reasonable precaution.

THE BOTTOM LINE: Electric blankets should be used with caution, especially during the first trimester.

Electrolysis

Electrolysis is the permanent removal of hair by killing the hair follicle with an electric current. Electrolysis can be used to remove hair from any part of the body.

CONCERNS: The American Electrology Association has published guidelines for electrolysis during pregnancy. The guidelines do not recommend performing electrolysis on the abdomen throughout the entire pregnancy or on the breasts and in the bikini area during third trimester pregnancy. Nevertheless, no published scientific literature examines the effects of electrolysis during pregnancy. No cases of birth defects or pregnancy complications attributed to electrolysis have been reported.

THE BOTTOM LINE: If you elect to have electrolysis during pregnancy, make sure to use a licensed electrologist who is aware that you are pregnant. Facial electrolysis is probably safe, but since this is an elective procedure and other methods are available for hair removal, consider waiting until after you deliver for electrolysis on your breasts, abdomen, or bikini area.

Enemas

Enemas are introduced into the colon via the rectum to cause a bowel movement. They can be made from a variety of substances.

CONCERNS: Because some people have suggested the use of enemas to stimulate the induction of labor, there is concern that use during pregnancy could possibly cause preterm labor. Traditionally, enemas have been administered routinely upon admission to a hospital's labor and delivery area to prevent the passage of stool during the pushing stage and fecal contamination of the baby. The few studies that have looked at enema use in relation to cervical ripening and the induction of labor have failed to find a benefit to using enemas for this purpose. Another study looked at the routine use of enemas in early labor and its relation to infection and also found no clear benefits.

Constipation is a common problem during pregnancy, and you might be tempted to use an enema for relief. However, the best treatment for constipation is to increase the amount of fiber in your diet. Enemas can cause dehydration due to the rapid loss of material from the colon.

THE BOTTOM LINE: Although the use of enemas probably is safe, generally there is little need for them during pregnancy. If you require one for a specific medical condition, you need not worry. If you desire to have one in early labor, feel free to do so, but keep well hydrated.

Energy drinks

Two types of beverages are touted as energy drinks. One is the creamy, high-calorie nutritional drink used by hospitals and nursing homes to provide liquid meals for those who cannot eat. Brand names include Boost® and Ensure®, and they are now available in most consumer markets. The second type of energy drink is high in caffeine and sugar to provide a jolt of energy. These drinks also contain a variety of other substances, including herbs, such as guarana (see Guarana), kava kava, and ma huang; amino acids, such as taurine (see Taurine); and other chemicals. Brand names include Adrenaline Rush®, Amp®, Extreme Ripped Force®, Red Bull®, Speed Stack®, and Venom®.

CONCERNS: It is probably not wise to substitute high-calorie drinks for meals, pregnant or not. Although they do provide calories, vitamins, and minerals, they are lacking in fiber and are no substitute for a well-balanced diet.

Concern over caffeine (see Caffeine) and other herbs should make you wary of many of these drinks during pregnancy. Although it appears to be safe to consume 300 milligrams (mg) caffeine or less per day during pregnancy, most health care providers still advised moderation. Eight ounces of Ensure® contain 10 mg caffeine; high-energy drinks can contain as much as 100 mg caffeine.

Taurine, a nonessential amino acid found in meat, dairy, and seafood, is added to many of these beverages to boost energy. There are no known safe limits of supplemental taurine during pregnancy, and no studies have examined the interactions of taurine with other chemicals. Similarly, d-glucurono-γ-lactone or glucuronolactone, a metabolite of glucose, is added to many of these drinks, and while there are no known harmful effects, safe levels of this compound are not known.

Further, some of these products are categorized as food supplements and are not regulated by the U.S. Food and Drug Administration. Thus, there is no guarantee of the strength, purity, or safety of these products. You should inform your health care provider if you are taking any nutritional supplements.

THE BOTTOM LINE: Since there is no good reason to consume these beverages during pregnancy, it is probably best to avoid them. If you feel an energy drink is necessary, carefully read the ingredients so that you know what you are consuming, and discuss individual ingredients with your OB/GYN.

Ensure®

Ensure® is a brand name for a creamy, high-calorie nutritional drink (see Energy drinks).

Epidural anesthesia

Epidural anesthesia (see Anesthetic, local) is a type of regional anesthesia. The technique involves placing a needle into the epidural space, the space between the vertebrae and the spinal canal, to introduce a small tube through which medications can be introduced that act to numb the nerves. Epidurals are generally used for labor analgesia and cesarean sections and are administered by an anesthesiologist or a nurse anesthetist.

CONCERNS: According to several studies, an association between labor epidural use and cesarean section was found. These results are now being disputed as more recent studies involving over 22,000 women have found no such association.

There is also concern over complications related to epidurals including risks of infection, spinal headache, drops in blood pressure, and temporary back soreness.

THE BOTTOM LINE: Epidurals are the most effective way to control pain during labor and are considered to be very safe.

Equal®

Equal® is a brand name for aspartame (*see* Aspartame; Artificial sweeteners).

Erythromycin

Erythromycin is an antibiotic (*see* Antibiotics, oral).

CONCERNS: No studies have shown an association between erythromycin use during pregnancy and birth defects. Erythromycin has been assigned a risk factor category of B (*see* Appendix 1).

THE BOTTOM LINE: Erythromycin is safe during pregnancy.

Esomeprazole

Esomeprazole, also known by the brand name Nexium®, is a type of antacid (*see* Antacids) that is classified as a proton pump inhibitor (PPI). PPIs work to block the secretion of acid from the cells of the stomach. This drug is used to treat the symptoms of gastroesophageal reflux disease (GERD).

CONCERNS: Because esomeprazole is a new drug, there have been no studies examining its effects on human pregnancy. However, studies in laboratory animals have not shown any harm during pregnancy. Esomeprazole has a risk factor category of B (*see* Appendix 1).

THE BOTTOM LINE: Due to the limited amount of data regarding the safety of this drug, esomeprazole is not recommended for use during pregnancy.

Essential oils

Essential oils are oils, generally derived from plants, that can be used for aromatherapy or topically in the form of massage oil, in a salve, or in a bath. In most cases, the oils are diluted prior to application to the skin. Examples of essential oils include grapefruit, lavender, lemon, orange, camomile, cedarwood, peppermint, rosemary, basil, caraway, cinnamon, sage, clove, and wintergreen. They have multiple uses, including treatment for morning sickness, swollen ankles, and headache.

CONCERNS: Therapists who use essential oils tend to err on the side of caution and may even suggest completely avoiding these oils during pregnancy. Those who use them will suggest waiting until after the first trimester (12 weeks) due to concern over miscarriage, as some are used to bring on menstruation.

No scientific studies document the safety of essential oils. One study showed that the use of aromatherapy during labor did reduce anxiety and the need for pain medication. There was one reported case of a camomile enema causing anaphylactic (severe allergic reaction) shock.

THE BOTTOM LINE: Little scientific data are available on the effects of these oils during pregnancy.

Evening primrose oil

Evening primrose oil (EPO) is oil rich in linoleic acid, which is an essential amino acid. It can be taken as a capsule by mouth or applied directly to the cervix or skin. It is commonly used for premenstrual syndrome, cervical ripening prior to labor, eczema, and arthritis.

CONCERNS: Since EPO is categorized as a food supplement, it is not regulated by the FDA. Thus, there is no guarantee of the strength, purity, or safety of EPO. You should inform your health care provider if you are taking any nutritional supplements. It is unknown whether this supplement is safe in pregnancy.

Several studies have looked at the effectiveness of inducing labor using EPO. Unfortunately, all of them have failed to find any benefit; one even found a higher risk of prolonged rupture of membranes, increased use of pitocin (a medication used to cause uterine labor contractions), and increased instrumented (needing to use forceps or a vacuum) deliveries.

THE BOTTOM LINE: Although probably safe, there appears to be little benefit to taking EPO during pregnancy.

Excedrin®

Excedrin® is a brand name for aspirin (*see* Aspirin; Pain relievers).

Exercise

The U.S. Department of Health and Human Services chooses to focus on a different goal each year to improve the nation's health. One focus for 2005 was to encourage more physical activity. This organization recommends that most adults should exercise 30 minutes per day. The American College of Obstetrics and Gynecology (ACOG) echoes this recommendation.

CONCERNS: Concern about exercise centers around the potential effects on the baby and the risks of injury to the mother.

In 1985, the ACOG recommended that you maintain your heart rate below 140 beats per minute (bpm) while exercising. In 1994, the revised Committee Opinion omitted any reference to heart rate during exercise, as there are no adequate studies examining the effects of maternal heart rates during exercise and fetal outcomes.

Currently the ACOG recommends 30 minutes or more of moderate exercise on most if not all days for most pregnant women. Regular exercise has been associated with prevention of gestational diabetes (diabetes related to pregnancy), controlling weight gain, and maternal well-being. Women at risk for preterm labor or who have an incompetent cervix (a cervix that dilates painlessly and prematurely), ruptured membranes, or bleeding are generally advised to limit their exercise.

Pregnancy results in several physiologic changes that may require you to adjust your usual routine. During pregnancy the amount of the hormone relaxin increases in the blood. Relaxin is a hormone produced by the reproductive tract during pregnancy. Its main role is to inhibit uterine contractions, soften the cervix, and dilate blood vessels. Relaxin also works on other tissues such as ligaments and can make it easier to strain muscles and ligaments while exercising. Listen to your body. If you are having pain, you may want to slow down. Limit exercise that involves supine positions (lying down) if you feel dizzy while in that position. Be careful to keep well hydrated and avoid becoming overheated, as this has been associated with preterm contractions produced during pregnancy. There is a theoretical risk that increases in your core body temperature in the first trimester caused by exercising could cause birth defects. However, studies have not shown any increase in core temperature with moderate exercise. As your body changes as your baby grows, you may find that you need to slow down or shorten your workouts.

Exercises with a high potential for abdominal trauma should be avoided, including ice hockey, soccer, and basketball. Exercises with risk of falling should be avoided, including horseback riding (*see* Horseback riding), downhill skiing (*see* Skiing), biking (*see* Biking), and gymnastics. Finally, scuba diving (*see* Scuba diving) should be avoided because of the risk of decompression syndrome.

THE BOTTOM LINE: Although exercise is safe and is encouraged in most cases, use common sense and slow down if you are experiencing pain, contractions, dizziness, or vaginal bleeding. If you exercise with a trainer or take a class, you should inform her/him that you are pregnant so any necessary modifications can be discussed. Consider trying a pregnancy exercise class or workout. In general, it is not recommended that you start any new exercise routines while pregnant, but if you are already in a routine, it is healthy to continue with it. If you have any concerns, please discuss these with your OB/GYN.

Expectorants

Expectorants (*see* Cough and cold suppressants) are medications used to break up chest secretions. They may be sold over the counter or by prescription. Guaifenesin (*see* Guaifenesin) is the most common over-the-counter expectorant and is found in Benylin®, Cough-X®, and Robitussin®. Codeine (*see* Codeine) and hydrocodone are expectorants found in prescription medications.

CONCERNS: Most expectorants are assigned a risk factor category of B, C, or D (*see* Appendix 1).

THE BOTTOM LINE: Most expectorants appear to be safe in pregnancy. Discuss individual medications with your health care provider.

Extreme Ripped Force®

Extreme Ripped Force® is a brand name of an energy drink (*see* Energy drinks).

[F]

Fertilizer ⚠

Fertilizer is used to aid the growth of plants. Fertilizers can be derived from plant or animal sources. They generally contain nitrogen, phosphorus, and potassium, which plants need for growth. More than 54 million tons of commercial fertilizer are used in the United States every year.

CONCERNS: Improper use of fertilizers can cause contamination of soil and groundwater (*see* Tap water). Nitrogen can form nitrates (*see* Nitrates and nitrites) and contaminate drinking water. Fertilizers can also become contaminated with heavy metals, pesticides (*see* Pesticides), and bacteria such as *Salmonella* (*see Salmonella*). Little is known about the possible interactions between the chemicals that are contaminating our groundwater.

A recent study looked at fertilizer/pesticide combinations common to two separate regions in the United States and could find no association with pregnancy loss or congenital birth defects in laboratory mice and rats, even at high levels.

THE BOTTOM LINE: Improper handling of fertilizer is known to cause contamination of soil and groundwater. Not much is known about the effects of this contamination on human pregnancy.

Feta ⚠

Feta is a Greek-style cheese (*see* Cheese) that is generally made from goat's or sheep's milk but can also be made from cow's milk. It is cured and stored in a salty brine. Feta is considered to be a soft cheese.

CONCERNS: Since feta can be made from raw (unpasteurized) milk, caution should be used during pregnancy (*see* Unpasteurized cheeses). All cheese made in the United States is made only from pasteurized milk. The U.S. Food and Drug Administration allows the importation of raw-milk cheese into the United States only if the cheese is aged 60 days or more. The harmful bacteria die as a result of the aging process. Young cheese aged less than 60 days made from unpasteurized milk is not allowed into the country.

Even if the cheese you are eating is made from pasteurized milk, contamination of soft cheese with harmful bacteria such as *Listeria monocytogenes* (*see* Listeria) can occur. This bacterium can cause preterm labor and stillbirth during pregnancy. The Centers for Disease Control and Prevention (CDC) recommends avoiding all soft cheese, including feta, during pregnancy. The high sugar and moisture content of soft cheese is favorable for bacterial growth. The risk of contamination can be decreased, but not prevented, by keeping your refrigerator at 40°F/4.5°C or below; keeping your refrigerator clean; avoiding cross-contamination from countertops, cutting boards, and utensils; and not leaving cheese unrefrigerated for more than two hours.

THE BOTTOM LINE: The CDC recommends avoiding feta during pregnancy. Cooking this cheese until boiling/bubbling should eliminate any harmful bacteria.

Fexofenadine

Fexofenadine is an antihistamine (*see* Antihistamines). A brand name for this drug is Allegra®.

CONCERNS: Fexofenadine has been assigned a risk factor category of C (*see* Appendix 1). Fexofenadine should not be used for prolonged periods or at high doses close to term.

THE BOTTOM LINE: Fexofenadine is safe to take during pregnancy for short periods before the third trimester.

Fiber supplements

Fiber supplements are used in the treatment of constipation. They also may help to lower cholesterol levels and keep blood glucose levels more constant. They are sold under the brand names of Metamucil® and Citru-cel®. Fiber supplements can also be consumed in cereals and other foods that have fiber added to them. Fiber can be obtained from the diet from fruits, vegetables, and whole grains.

CONCERNS: Some women experience an increased rate of constipation during pregnancy that is due to increased hormonal levels that slow down the intestinal transit time; increased uterine size; changes in diet; prenatal vitamins (see Multivitamins), calcium supplements (see Calcium), and antacids (see Antacids); and changes in exercise patterns (see Exercise). Increasing your fiber and water intake, and not taking laxatives (see Laxatives), is considered to be the treatment of choice for constipation in pregnancy. However, fiber supplements can cause bloating, abdominal cramping, and flatulence, so add fiber slowly and drink plenty of water to minimize any side effects.

Most fiber supplements have been assigned a pregnancy risk factor category of B (see Appendix I).

THE BOTTOM LINE: Fiber supplements are considered to be safe during pregnancy. If you are adding fiber supplements to your diet, drink plenty of water.

Fish ⚠

Fish are generally broken down into two categories, fish and shellfish (see Shellfish). Fish have fins, backbones, and gills. Shellfish have shells. There are many varieties of fish, including tuna (see Tuna), shark, swordfish, salmon, and cod. Fish can be prepared in a variety of ways, including fried, broiled, grilled, marinated, and raw. Fish are high in protein and omega-3 fatty acids.

CONCERNS: A recent study involving over 9,000 pregnancies showed that women who ate no seafood during their pregnancies were more likely to have a child with a lower verbal intelligence as compared to women who ate 12 ounces of seafood per week. However, concern over mercury (see Methylmercury) levels and other toxins in certain species of fish has motivated the Environmental Protection Agency (EPA) and the U.S. Food and Drug Administration (FDA) to release guidelines on fish consumption for pregnant women and young children. Tuna, shark, swordfish, king mackerel, and tile fish (a.k.a. golden or white snapper) are known to have higher levels of methylmercury. Fish that are low in mercury include salmon, cod, pollock, catfish, shrimp, and flounder. The FDA recommends limiting fish high in mercury to two 6-ounce servings per week.

Due to concerns over pollutants, freshwater fish caught in local waters should be limited during pregnancy, as they are rarely monitored by the EPA. Polychlorinated biphenyls (PCBs) have been associated with decreased attention span, memory, and IQ levels. Bluefish, striped bass, salmon, pike, trout, and walleye from contaminated lakes and rivers may contain PCBs within their fat. Check with your local health department to see if the fish in your area are known to be polluted.

Sushi (*see* Sushi) and smoked fish (*see* Smoked fish) should also be consumed with caution during pregnancy. Sushi and smoked fish may be contaminated with *Listeria* (*see* Listeria) and *Campylobacter* (*see Campylobacter*). Raw fish may also contain parasites, such as tapeworms. Freezing the fish prior to consumption, which is often done for sushi, will kill adult parasitic worms but small eggs will persist, as well as hepatitis A and other viruses.

THE BOTTOM LINE: Certain fish have been found to contain high levels of mercury and should be limited during pregnancy. You can safely eat 12 ounces of *any* cooked fish per week. Sushi and smoked fish may be contaminated with bacteria, viruses, and parasites that can cause illness. Smoked fish that are cooked, canned, or shelf stable are safe to eat during pregnancy. That being said, fish contain many healthy nutrients that are important for you and your baby's health. Keep aware of changing recommendations.

Fish oil

Fish oil can be purchased in health food stores in a capsule form. This oil can also be consumed by eating fish. Fish oil is rich in omega-3 fatty acids, a healthy part of your diet. These fatty acids have been shown to decrease your risk of heart disease, hypertension, and stroke. Fish oil differs from cod liver oil (*see* Cod liver oil) in that it is not rich in Vitamins A (*see* Vitamin A) and D (*see* Vitamin D).

CONCERNS: A recent retrospective study found that women who consume fish at least once a week during the first 16 weeks of pregnancy have a lower risk of having a small baby and preterm labor compared to women who ate no fish at all. Another study found that consumption of omega-3 fatty acids was associated with decreased rates of depression during the third trimester and the postpartum period.

As a result of concerns over mercury toxicity, some people may look to supplement their diets with fish oil. Unless it is clear which fish are used to produce fish oil, it is possible that the oils could contain high levels of methylmercury (*see* Methylmercury).

The consumption of certain oils can cause diarrhea and possibly preterm labor. If you experience diarrhea from fish oil, it is probably wise to decrease the amount that you are taking.

THE BOTTOM LINE: Fish oil appears to be safe and may even be beneficial during pregnancy.

Flagyl® *See* Metronidazole.

Flaxseed

Flaxseed is a seed that contains calcium (*see* Calcium), iron, niacin (*see* Niacin), phosphorus, and Vitamin E (*see* Vitamin E). It also contains high quantities of omega-3 and omega-6 fatty acids and fiber. It is the source of linseed oil, which is used in paint, varnishes, linoleums, and inks, and is also found in many baked goods. It can be purchased as a seed or pre-ground, or in the form of flaxseed oil. Some people supplement their diets with flaxseed to ensure they are consuming enough omega-3 fatty acids without risking the mercury (*see* Mercury; Methylmercury) found in fish or Vitamin A (*see* Vitamin A) in cod liver oil (*see* Cod liver oil).

Flaxseed may also have some estrogenic effects. Because estrogen is a hormone that is produced in reduced amounts after menopause, some women supplement their diets with flaxseed to relieve symptoms related to menopause. A few studies have promoted flaxseed as healthful and useful in preventing heart disease, kidney disease, and menopausal symptoms and in the treatment of constipation.

CONCERNS: Providers who prescribe flaxseed caution against its use in pregnancy secondary to any possible estrogenic effects that may affect the growing baby. Several studies using laboratory rats did not show any teratogenic (causing birth defects) effects due to flaxseed, but did note some secondary sex abnormalities in the rats exposed to flaxseed in utero.

THE BOTTOM LINE: Not much is known about the effects of flaxseed use during pregnancy. Due to evidence in laboratory animals that it may cause some issues with secondary sexual development, it is probably best to avoid during pregnancy.

Flea and tick medication

Several preparations are used to treat ticks and fleas on domestic pets. These include collars and other medications that are applied directly to your pet's fur or skin, such as Frontline® and Advantage®. Flea and tick collars are placed on the cat or dog for an extended period of time (usually several months). The insecticide within the collar is released and spreads evenly across the pet's skin. Topical medications persist on the pet for varying lengths of time. Repeated (monthly) application may be required. If a tick or flea bites the pet, it will ingest the insecticide and die.

CONCERNS: Women exposed to household insecticides (see Insecticides, home use) are 1.5 times more likely to have a child with a birth defect. The most common defects noted were neural tube defects, facial defects, and limb defects. The greatest risk appears to be with exposure during the first trimester and with prolonged exposure. A recent study showed an association between using flea/tick collars with pediatric brain tumors. This risk was highest for women who applied the flea collars themselves.

THE BOTTOM LINE: The safest thing to do is to avoid all insecticides throughout your pregnancy and especially during the first trimester. There appears to be an increased risk of birth defects with early and prolonged exposure. Avoid applying collars or topical preparations yourself to decrease your exposure to the chemicals.

Flu vaccination

The flu vaccination is an intramuscular vaccination used to cause immunity against a specific strain of the influenza virus.

CONCERNS: Vaccinations or immunizations (*see* Immunizations) are medications, many of which can cross the placenta. Currently the Centers for Disease Control and Prevention recommends the flu vaccine for all pregnant women, regardless of trimester. There has been an association between influenza infection during pregnancy and schizophrenia in the offspring, and it has been postulated that vaccination of all pregnant women will reduce the incidence of schizophrenia.

There have been some concerns about the mercury used in the vaccine (*see* Mercury), but the amounts used are extremely small and are not known to cause any adverse pregnancy outcomes.

THE BOTTOM LINE: The flu vaccination is safe in pregnancy.

Fluconazole

Fluconazole is the antifungal found in Diflucan® (*see* Antifungal medications, oral and topical).

CONCERNS: Fluconazole has been assigned a risk factor category of C (*see* Appendix 1).

THE BOTTOM LINE: Fluconazole is considered to be safe in pregnancy.

Fluoride

Fluoride is a naturally occurring element that helps the body to retain calcium for strong bones and teeth. It can be found in organ meats, fish, apples, and eggs (*see* Eggs). Sodium fluoride may be added to drinking water and certain toothpastes, and may be taken as a supplement to reduce the risk of tooth decay.

There is controversy over the issue of fluoride supplementation during pregnancy. Studies have shown that fluoride can cross the placenta, and since 1966 the U.S. Food and Drug Administration has banned the use of advertising and labeling of fluoride supplements for prenatal use. One study has demonstrated a link between fluoride supplementation and attention deficit hyperactivity disorder (ADHD) in children.

Other researchers have claimed that fluoride supplementation could help reduce the risk of birth defects, including neural tube defects. Some studies have reported that fluoride supplementation is completely safe during pregnancy.

THE BOTTOM LINE: The safe doses of prenatal fluoride have not been established. Due to this and the conflicting literature, it is probably best to avoid fluoride supplementation during pregnancy. However, routine use in toothpaste and in drinking water appears to be safe.

Foie gras ⚠

Foie gras is the liver of a goose or duck that has been force-fed a high-fat diet over four to five months. The fowl are not permitted to exercise during this period of time. After the livers are removed, they are generally soaked in milk, water, or port, and then marinated and seasoned. The livers are then baked. This process produces a smooth and rich texture that is considered a delicacy.

CONCERNS: A study in 2001 by the Food Safety and Inspection Service of the United States Department of Agriculture (FSIS/USDA) determined that many pregnant women were either not aware of the dangers of certain foods or did not handle these foods properly in the home. It is important to know that you are at risk for several food-borne illnesses that can be contracted through prepared meats (see Deli meats, cooked and uncooked) during pregnancy.

Foie gras is susceptible to Listeria (see Listeria) from contamination by meat slicers, cutting boards (see Cutting boards), knives, and refrigerators. Even if the food is properly refrigerated, this bacterium may still be present. Although you won't be completely eliminating the risks, the USDA recommends that precooked meats should be properly stored below 40°F/4.5°C and should be thrown away if they have an expired freshness date. Cooking foie gras until steaming hot will ensure that all harmful parasites and bacteria are killed. There is also some concern over the amount of vitamin A (see Vitamin A) found in liver (see Codfish liver oil). Although concern over high intakes of vitamin A is warranted, foie gras is usually served in very small portions so the vitamin A content would not usually be an issue.

THE BOTTOM LINE: Properly cooked foie gras is safe.

Folic acid ☑

Folic acid, also known as folate, folacin, and Vitamin B_9, is a water-soluble B vitamin found in leafy green vegetables, liver, lentils, chick peas, strawberries, oranges, kidney beans, and enriched grains.

CONCERNS: Studies have been able to show a clear association between adequate folic acid intake and the reduction of neural tube defects. Due to this association, physicians have recommended supplementation for women while trying to become pregnant and during early pregnancy, when these defects can occur.

The Centers for Disease Control and Prevention (CDC) recommends 400 micrograms (mcg) or 0.4 milligrams (mg) folic acid every day. This should be taken for one month prior to conception. During pregnancy, you should increase your dose to 600 to 800 mcg daily. Many prenatal vitamins contain these doses; some contain up to 1,000 mcg. This vitamin is water soluble, so if you take more than is needed, your body will flush out the rest. Your doctor may recommend that you take a higher dose if you have certain risk factors or if you have had a prior pregnancy affected by a neural tube defect or take certain medications.

THE BOTTOM LINE: Multiple studies have shown the beneficial effects of folic acid during pregnancy. Stick to the CDC's recommendations to achieve its full benefit.

Food additives ⚠

A food additive is any ingredient added to food for flavor; to change the quality or color; or to preserve or add to its nutritional value. Examples of food additives include artificial sweeteners (*see* Artificial sweeteners), BHA/BHT (*see* BHA/BHT), caffeine (*see* Caffeine), food coloring (*see* Artificial coloring), MSG (*see* MSG), nitrates and nitrites (*see* Nitrates and nitrites), Vitamin A (*see* Vitamin A), and Vitamin C (*see* Vitamin C).

CONCERNS: The U.S. Food and Drug Administration evaluates many food additives and may classify them as generally recognized as safe or GRAS. The GRAS list contains hundreds of food additives. The GRAS classification means that the additive has been shown to be safe under conditions of its intended use. Examples of additives on the GRAS list include salt, vinegar, guar gum, MSG, Vitamin A, Vitamin C, BHA/BHT, and caffeine.

Keep in mind that some of the additives on the GRAS list may be dangerous during pregnancy if taken in large amounts. Examples of this include Vitamin A and caffeine.

Even when the U.S. FDA declares a food additive as safe for use in food, public opinion can make us worry about the safety of a food additive. This appears to be the case with aspartame (*see* Aspartame). Studies show that aspartame does not cross the placenta and it appears to be safe in pregnancy.

Several food additives have been associated with health risks and should probably be avoided, especially during pregnancy. These include certain artificial colorings, nitrates and nitrites, and saccharin.

THE BOTTOM LINE: Avoidance of processed foods, especially during pregnancy and early childhood, will help decrease the amounts of food additives that you ingest. Quickly reading the labels of food you buy will help you avoid unwanted additives in your diet.

Foot massage *See* Massage. ✅

Frontline® 🚫

Frontline® is a brand name of tick and flea medication for pets (*see* Flea and tick medication).

Fungi ✅

Fungi are organisms that include mushrooms, molds, and yeast. They are often used in cooking, but can also cause disease.

CONCERNS: Some fungi are known to cause disease in humans, including ringworm, allergies, athlete's foot, and vaginal yeast infections. Although bothersome, most fungal infections are not dangerous and are easily treated with antifungal agents (*see* Antifungal medications, oral and topical).

Molds are responsible for many allergy symptoms (*see* Allergy medications) and asthma (*see* Asthma) exacerbations.

THE BOTTOM LINE: Most fungi are not dangerous to a pregnancy. Mushrooms and yeast used in baked goods are safe to consume during pregnancy.

Gardasil®

Gardasil® is a new vaccination made by Merck & Co. that protects women from four types of human papillomavirus (HPV). These four virus types account for 70 percent of cervical cancers and 90 percent of genital wart cases. The vaccines are given in three doses over a six-month period. The vaccine is currently being given to girls and women who are between the ages of 9 and 26.

CONCERNS: Currently the vaccination is not recommended for women who are pregnant or are trying to conceive during the six-month vaccination period. Merck & Co. have started a pregnancy registry to look for any pregnancy problems. Despite these concerns, no animal studies have ever shown any reproductive problems with Gardasil®. Gardasil® has been assigned a pregnancy risk factor category of B (*see* Appendix 1).

THE BOTTOM LINE: There have been no adverse effects in women who have been inadvertently vaccinated, but Gardasil® is not currently recommended during pregnancy.

Gardening

According to the National Gardening Association, gardening in the United States is at an all-time high, with 85 million households participating in lawn and garden activities.

CONCERNS: Gardening puts you at risk for *Toxoplasmosis* (*see Toxoplasmosis*). *Toxoplasmosis gondii* is a parasite that can be spread through the feces of cats (*see* Cats; Litter boxes) and can also infect birds. If you do your gardening in soil that is visited by cats or birds, you run the risk of getting this parasite. Keep in mind that many people have been exposed to *Toxoplasmosis* during childhood and are immune. However, if you are not immune and contract this disease during pregnancy, you are at risk for preterm labor, miscarriage, and certain birth defects. You can avoid getting this parasite by wearing gloves while you garden, washing your hands carefully afterward, and avoiding touching your face with your gloves.

You may also be more sensitive to the effects of the sun during pregnancy. A good sunscreen, hat, and protective clothing will help reduce the risks of sun exposure (*see* Sun exposure).

Avoid the use of herbicides and pesticides during pregnancy (*see* Herbicides; Pesticides). Women who use pesticides during pregnancy are 1.5 more times likely to have a child with a birth defect.

Use fertilizer only as directed to reduce the risk of contamination of soil and groundwater (*see* Fertilizer).

Finally, most areas of the United States have been affected by the West Nile virus, which is transmitted through the bite of infected mosquitoes. The insect repellent DEET (*see* DEET; Insecticides, home use) is considered to be safe in pregnancy and should be used, as the risks of DEET use appear to be less than that of West Nile virus. Be careful to use as directed to limit your exposure to DEET.

THE BOTTOM LINE: With a little planning and protective gear, gardening is safe.

Gas Relief®

Gas Relief® is a brand name of simethicone (*see* Simethicone).

Gas-X®

Gas-X® is a brand name of Simethicone (*see* Simethicone).

Ginkgo biloba

Ginkgo biloba is made from the dried leaf of the ginkgo biloba plant. Clinical evidence supports its use for the treatment of age-associated memory impairment.

CONCERNS: One study demonstrated that colchicine, an active ingredient found in ginkgo biloba, was isolated in human placental blood from women taking ginkgo during pregnancy. Colchicine is used in the treatment of gout. Studies on the use of colchicine during pregnancy are limited in number. No birth defects have been noted in women who were exposed to this drug during pregnancy, but some teratogenic (birth-defect-causing) effects were seen at high doses in laboratory animals. As a result of this information, colchicine has been assigned a risk factor category of D (*see* Appendix 1).

Another known side effect of ginkgo biloba is that it can make it harder for blood to clot; thus, this herbal supplement should be avoided during pregnancy. Despite these worries, ginkgo biloba has been given a pregnancy risk factor category of C (*see* Appendix 1).

Since ginkgo biloba is categorized as a food supplement, it is not regulated by the U.S. Food and Drug Administration. Thus, there is no guarantee of the strength, purity, or safety of this product. You should inform your health care provider if you are taking any nutritional supplements.
THE BOTTOM LINE: Until more is known about the effects of this herbal supplement, there is initial evidence that ginkgo biloba should be avoided during pregnancy.

Ginseng

Ginseng is a plant found in widespread areas. Its root can be boiled and used for a tea (*see* Herb tea) or soup or ground and placed in a capsule. Ginseng is taken to treat a variety of conditions, most commonly to improve stamina, for relief of stress and fatigue, and as an anticancer drug.
CONCERNS: One retrospective report demonstrated that a woman taking large doses of ginseng had an infant with enlarged testes and abnormal secondary sex hair growth. A study from China has demonstrated birth defects in laboratory rats that were given ginseng during pregnancy.

Since ginseng is categorized as a food supplement, it is not regulated by the Food and Drug Administration. Thus, there is no guarantee of the strength, purity, or safety of this product. You should inform your health care provider if you are taking any nutritional supplements.

THE BOTTOM LINE: Preliminary studies indicate that there may be an increased risk of birth defects if ginseng is taken during pregnancy. Therefore, until more is known, this herb should be avoided during pregnancy.

Glucosamine

Glucosamine is a substance naturally produced by the body and is necessary for the formation of tendons, ligaments, skin, bones, and membranes. Glucosamine sulfate can be taken as a nutritional supplement and is used to promote cartilage growth and as an anti-inflammatory agent. It is commonly used for the treatment of osteoarthritis.

CONCERNS: Studies revealed changes in neonatal metabolism as a result of this supplement during pregnancy. Since glucosamine is categorized as a food supplement, it is not regulated by the Food and Drug Administration. Thus, there is no guarantee of the strength, purity, or safety of this product. You should inform your health care provider if you are taking any nutritional supplements.

THE BOTTOM LINE: Although its effects have not been fully evaluated during pregnancy, the Arthritis Association cautions against the use of glucosamine sulfate during pregnancy.

Glycolic peels

In a glycolic peel, the chemical glycolic acid is applied to the face to remove dead surface skin from the top layer of the face. Advocates believe that glycolic peels result in smoother and softer skin, with the reduction of fine lines and age spots.

CONCERNS: Since the glycolic acid is applied to the skin for several minutes, there is some concern as to how much is absorbed from the skin into the bloodstream.

THE BOTTOM LINE: Not much is known about glycolic peels during pregnancy. Glycolic acid appears to be safe and is applied to the skin for short periods of time (usually less than 10 minutes). Glycolic peels are probably safe, but use caution until more is known.

Green tea *See* Tea. ⚠

Guaifenesin ☑

Guaifenesin is an expectorant (*see* Expectorants; Cough and cold suppressants) that acts to decrease coughs. It is the most commonly used over-the-counter expectorant and can be found in Benylin®, Cough-X®, and Robitussin®.

CONCERNS: Studies have shown no association between guaifenesin and birth defects. Guaifenesin has been assigned a risk factor category of C (*see* Appendix 1).

THE BOTTOM LINE: Guaifenesin is considered to be safe in pregnancy.

Guarana ⚠

Guarana is a shrub found in the Amazon. The seeds are dried, roasted, and then made into a paste that is used in foods, drinks, and medicines. As a medicine, guarana has many uses, including as an astringent, a stimulant, to prevent cardiovascular disease, and to treat diarrhea.

CONCERNS: One of the active ingredients in guarana is a form of caffeine (*see* Caffeine). It has been estimated that 5 grams of guarana seeds contain 250 milligrams of caffeine. Some guarana preparations contain as much as two to three times the caffeine found in coffee or tea. Guarana also contains other chemicals, such as theobromine and theophylline. Theobromine is similar to caffeine. Theophylline is a drug with a risk factor C (*see* Appendix 1) that is used to treat asthma (*see* Asthma) and other respiratory diseases.

Since guarana is categorized as a food supplement, it is not regulated by the Food and Drug Administration. Thus, there is no guarantee of the strength, purity, or safety of this product. You should inform your health care provider if you are taking any nutritional supplements.

THE BOTTOM LINE: As with other forms of caffeine, caution should be used with guarana during pregnancy.

Hair dyes

Hair dyes include all hair treatments used for changing the color of hair. CONCERNS: The U.S. Food and Drug Administration recommends that until conclusive evidence is available, pregnant women may want to proceed with caution when using hair dyes.

Low levels of hair dye have been found to be absorbed into the skin and are then excreted into the urine. These low levels have not been associated with any adverse fetal outcomes. Also, there have been no reported negative outcomes from women who have had their hair dyed during pregnancy.

THE BOTTOM LINE: Hair dye has not been associated with any adverse fetal outcomes, but you should use caution until there is more evidence documenting its safety. If you choose to dye your hair while pregnant, consider using a technique that involves the shortest possible time of exposure to the chemicals used and waiting until after the first trimester.

Haldol®

Haldol® is a brand name for haloperidol (*see* Psychiatric medications).

Head lice

Head lice are parasitic insects (*see* Parasites) that live on human blood from the scalp. They most commonly affect school-age children and their families, as they are easily spread by close contact.

CONCERNS: Concern over head lice centers around treatment issues. Medicated shampoos used to get rid of head lice are not recommended for children under the age of two, and several shampoos and herbal remedies are considered to be contraindicated in pregnancy.

Nit combing is the treatment of choice in pregnancy. Nits are the eggs of the lice, deposited on the hair strands. However, if combing does not work, both permethrin, sold under the brand name Nix®, and lindane, sold under the brand name Kwell®, have a risk factor category of B (*see* Appendix 1) and are considered to be safe in pregnancy. The use of lindane is controversial; despite the fact that lindane has a risk factor of B, some feel that it should not be used in pregnancy due to a risk of central nervous system toxicity in the treated individual. To control a head lice infestation, it is necessary to treat family contacts and take environmental measures, including washing all clothes and bed linens in 130°F/55°C water and vacuuming.

THE BOTTOM LINE: Although not dangerous in and of themselves, head lice are annoying and can spread to others. Nit combing is the treatment method of choice. However, if this is not satisfactory, many medicated shampoos may be safely used during pregnancy. Consider trying olive oil if nit combing is unsuccessful and you desire to avoid medications.

Health clubs ⚠

A health club is any facility that has exercise or spa equipment.

CONCERNS: Continuing to exercise (*see* Exercise) during pregnancy is strongly encouraged, as new studies have demonstrated the many potential benefits of exercise. With these new studies, attention has also been turned to the potential dangers in health clubs including saunas (*see* Saunas), hot tubs (*see* Hot tubs), and swimming pools (*see* Pools).

Concern over the use of saunas and hot tubs has centered on the possibility of increasing maternal core body temperature (CBT). Numerous studies have made an association between elevated temperatures and the increased incidence of neural tube defects and miscarriages.

Further study suggests a significant or greater association when your CBT rises to 102.5°F/39.2°C. Some researchers have suggested that if a pregnant woman's CBT becomes that high, she would feel uncomfortable and get out of the tub. Taking a hot shower does not usually result in an increased CBT.

There also exists some concern over chlorinated pools (*see* Chlorine). A few studies have found that a group of by-products of chlorine, trihalomethanes (THMs), can be found in water treated with chlorine and is associated with low birth weight and fetal birth defects, such as neural tube defects. THMs can be absorbed through the skin or lungs. It is unclear as to what levels are dangerous during pregnancy. Other studies have not found this association. Chlorine can also break down into chloroform, which may also cause harm during a pregnancy. The Environmental Protection Agency has set up standards to monitor these levels and is continuing to do research on this issue. Swimming during periods of low use appears to be associated with lower THM levels.

THE BOTTOM LINE: Continue to exercise if you are having a normal pregnancy. Discuss exercise guidelines with your health care provider. Avoid the use of saunas and hot tubs during pregnancy. Consider using the pool when it is less crowded, and rinse off any chlorine following your swim.

Heavy lifting

Heavy lifting is defined as lifting objects greater than 25 pounds.

CONCERNS: Physically demanding work has been linked to preterm labor, preeclampsia (hypertension, protein in the urine, and swelling), and low birth weight.

During pregnancy, the amount of the hormone relaxin in the blood increases. Relaxin is a hormone produced by the reproductive tract during pregnancy. Its main role is to inhibit uterine contractions, soften the cervix, and dilate blood vessels. Relaxin also works on other tissues such as ligaments and can make it easier to strain muscles and ligaments while exercising. To try to prevent injuries from occurring, use caution when doing physical labor. The American Medical Women's Association suggests that risk management programs include a weight-lifting restriction of 25 pounds (10 to 12 kilograms) for pregnant women.

THE BOTTOM LINE: Repeated heavy lifting during pregnancy should be avoided due to concerns of preterm labor, back pain, and other potential pregnancy complications.

Hemorrhoid medications

Many pregnant women develop hemorrhoids (inflammation and dilatation of veins in the rectum) during pregnancy. Hemorrhoid medications are used to treat the symptoms of hemorrhoids. Treatments for hemorrhoids include sitz baths, dietary changes, and over-the-counter creams and ointments. Some common hemorrhoid medications include Anusol®, Preparation H®, and Tucks®.

CONCERNS: Anusol®, Preparation H®, and Tucks® are considered to be safe for use during pregnancy. These medications are generally used along with more conservative therapies, such as sitz baths.

Some hemorrhoids require surgical management, but since they can improve after pregnancy, most providers will reevaluate the hemorrhoids after delivery.

THE BOTTOM LINE: Most over-the-counter hemorrhoid medications are safe for use during pregnancy.

Henna tattoos

Henna tattoos use henna, a naturally occurring pigment that is applied to the skin to create a temporary skin decoration or tattoo. Over thousands of years many women have applied henna tattoos to their pregnant abdomens in order to bring good luck to their pregnancies.

CONCERNS: Some dermatologists caution that skin may be more sensitive during pregnancy and you may be at risk for a reaction to the dye. There are two types of henna commonly used: Natural henna has a reddish brown color and lasts for about four weeks. Black henna contains para-phenylendiamine that may cause a bad skin reaction including blisters and burns and should be avoided.

THE BOTTOM LINE: Henna tattoos appear to be completely safe during pregnancy. If you are concerned about skin sensativity you can test a small area before getting a larger tattoo. Stick to natural henna and stay clear of black henna.

Herb tea ⚠

Herb teas are made by steeping herbs, flowers (petals, leaves, and/or stems), and/or spices in boiling water. They are commonly thought to have relaxing, calming, and medicinal properties.

CONCERNS: Since herbs are categorized as food supplements, they are not regulated by the U.S. Food and Drug Administration (FDA). Thus, there is no guarantee of the strength, purity, or safety of these products. You should inform your health care provider if you are taking any herbal supplements.

High doses of some herbs have been known to cause side effects such as diarrhea, vomiting, and heart palpitations. According to the FDA, commercially prepared teas in moderate amounts appear to be safe. If the ingredients are considered to be safe as foods (cinnamon, citrus peel, mint, ginger, lemon balm, and rose hip), they are assumed to be safe in teas. Use caution if you are making your own teas from raw bulk herbs.

Many herbal tea mixtures are sold as "pregnancy" teas to promote uterine and pregnancy health. Examples of herbal teas recommended during pregnancy include camomile, cinnamon, dandelion, lavender, lemon balm, nettle, red raspberry leaf, rose hips, spearmint, stevia, and wild oats. Some herbal teas are used to induce labor. They include anise, beth root, black cohosh, blue cohosh, borage, cramp bark, dill, lobelia, nettle, red raspberry, spikenard, and squaw vine. Use caution with these teas prior to term.

THE BOTTOM LINE: Commercially prepared herbal teas appear to be safe. Teas made from ingredients that are considered to be safe foods are safe in pregnancy. Use some caution with homemade teas from raw bulk herbs until more is known about any adverse effects during pregnancy.

Herbicides ⚠

Herbicides are chemicals that are used to kill weeds. Commonly used herbicides in the United States include atrazine, cyanazine, and metolachlor. Herbicides are sold under the brand names of Roundup®, Surlan®, and Vantage®.

CONCERNS: Herbicide use can cause contamination of groundwater and ultimately our drinking water. Because of this, studies examining the effects of herbicides in drinking water have been performed. One study that examined the effects of low levels of herbicides in the drinking water of pregnant mice showed a 20 percent increase in failed pregnancies.

A study examining the pregnant population of a farming community in the United States has shown an association between herbicides in the water and intrauterine growth restriction (low birth weight). The Environmental Protection Agency (EPA) regulates the chemicals found in public drinking water through testing, reporting, and public notification. The EPA does not monitor private well water. It considers atrazine, cyanazine, and metolachlor to be possible carcinogens. It is working to reduce the production and use of these chemicals both within the United States and internationally.

Other studies have shown that low levels of herbicides can cause fetal death and abnormalities in laboratory mice and frogs.

THE BOTTOM LINE: Low levels of herbicides have been found to cause fetal death and congenital abnormalities in both laboratory mice and frogs. Preventive measures should be taken when using herbicides during pregnancy. Use good ventilation and wear gloves when necessary. If you live in an area with high levels of herbicide use, contact the EPA for information and test your drinking water if it comes from a well, or used bottled water.

Herbs, medicinal

Medicinal herbs are plants that are used for medicinal purposes. They can be bought in several forms, including dried leaves, powders, capsules, and tablets. Examples of medicinal herbs include Echinacea (*see* Echinacea) and ginkgo biloba (*see* Ginkgo biloba).

CONCERNS: Estimates state that 50 to 75 percent of Americans use some form of alternative medicine, and $4.3 billion per year is spent on herbal supplements in this country. Despite this, most herbal supplements have not been studied with regard to their effects on pregnancy.

Since medicinal herbs are categorized as food supplements, they are not regulated by the U.S. Food and Drug Administration. Thus, there is no guarantee of the strength, purity, or safety of these products. You should inform your health care provider if you are taking any medicinal herbs.

THE BOTTOM LINE: Individual herbs should be researched prior to consumption during pregnancy. If there is no good information regarding their safety in pregnancy, which is often the case, it is probably safest to avoid their use.

Herpes

Herpes is a viral infection. There are two types, herpes simplex virus (HSV) I and HSV II. HSV I, or oral herpes, is characterized by cold sores near the mouth; HSV II is responsible for genital herpes. However, it is possible to have a genital lesion from HSV I and vice versa. Both types of the virus can be transmitted through direct contact. HSV is one of the most common viral sexually transmitted infections (STIs).

CONCERNS: Primary HSV infections or newly acquired HSV I can be transmitted to the fetus, cause preterm labor, and possibly cause birth defects. If you have a first outbreak of HSV during pregnancy, your health care provider may perform blood tests and prescribe antiviral medication. During recurrent infections, the mother has some protective antibodies that are passed to the fetus. The main concern with a recurrent outbreak is regarding the mode of delivery if an active lesion is present. In both primary and recurrent HSV, if you have an active genital lesion at the time of delivery, you may be advised to have a cesarean section to reduce the risk of transmission to the fetus.

If you have a history of HSV, your health care provider may suggest that you take prophylactic doses of antiviral medications during the third trimester of your pregnancy, to try to prevent an outbreak near delivery.

THE BOTTOM LINE: Herpes is a common viral infection. Primary HSV is worrisome during pregnancy and may have harmful effects on the baby. Both primary and recurrent HSV infection near the time of delivery may result in the need for delivery by cesarean section. Taking prophylactic antiviral medications may be beneficial in reducing the risk of an outbreak prior to delivery.

High altitudes ⚠️

High altitude is generally regarded as greater than 5,000 feet. Many women who are pregnant either live at high altitudes or plan vacations in these areas.

CONCERNS: Pregnancy at high altitude has been associated with smaller babies, preeclampsia (hypertension, protein in the urine, and swelling), and preterm labor.

If you are visiting an area that has a high altitude, be aware of the symptoms of altitude sickness. These symptoms include insomnia, fatigue, headache, nausea, and vomiting. Try to keep well hydrated and limit activity if you feel dizzy or are short of breath.

THE BOTTOM LINE: If you reside at high altitude, you are likely to have a normal pregnancy but do appear to be at increased risk for having a small baby and developing preeclampsia. Your health care provider should be able to look for these problems throughout your pregnancy. Short visits to high altitudes are safe if you are having a healthy pregnancy, but please be sure to keep hydrated and look for signs of problems.

High-heeled shoes ☑️

High-heeled shoes generally have heels of two or more inches.

CONCERNS: It is often recommended that you wear low-heeled shoes during pregnancy. Flat shoes and high-heeled shoes can cause back strain and lead to back pain. There is also a theoretical concern that high heels can make it easier for you to lose your balance and fall.

THE BOTTOM LINE: High heels are safe to wear during pregnancy. There is some evidence that wearing high-heeled shoes can increase your risk of foot, knee, and back pain.

⚠

Hollandaise sauce

Hollandaise sauce is made from butter, egg yolks (*see* Eggs), and lemon juice. It is a thick and creamy sauce that is served with vegetables, fish, and egg dishes, such as eggs Benedict. It is cooked over a double boiler and may contain undercooked eggs.

CONCERNS: Since the eggs are not fully cooked, there is a possibility that they could contain a bacterium called *Salmonella* (*see Salmonella*). *Salmonella* can cause diarrhea, fever, and abdominal pain. It is most dangerous in people who have a weakened immune system. Women who are pregnant do not appear to be at an increased risk of getting *Salmonella*. However, one type of this bacterium can cross the placenta and cause miscarriage, stillbirth, and preterm labor.

THE BOTTOM LINE: You should avoid Hollandaise sauce unless it is made with pasteurized eggs or from a commercially prepared mix. Cooking eggs to 165°F/74°C will destroy *Salmonella*. Wash your hands and utensils frequently to avoid cross-contamination when cooking with eggs.

Homemade ice cream

⚠

Ice cream is a frozen dessert made from milk, cream, sweeteners, and sometimes eggs (*see* Eggs). Other ingredients, such as chocolate, nuts, and fruit, may also be added.

CONCERNS: Since the eggs in homemade ice cream are not cooked, there is a possibility that they could contain a bacterium called *Salmonella* (*see Salmonella*). *Salmonella* can cause diarrhea, fever, and abdominal pain. It is most dangerous in people who have a weakened immune system. Women who are pregnant do not appear to be at an increased risk of getting *Salmonella*. However, one type of this bacterium can cross the placenta and cause miscarriage, stillbirth, and preterm labor. Ice cream made with unpasteurized milk could be contaminated with *Listeria* (*see Listeria*) or *Campylobacter* (*see Campylobacter*). Pregnant women are 20 times more likely to get listeriosis than other healthy adults. Infected pregnant women may have symptoms similar to the flu, such as fever and muscle aches, and infection may lead to preterm labor and even stillbirth. *Campylobacter* can cause miscarriage, preterm labor, and stillbirth.

THE BOTTOM LINE: You should avoid homemade ice cream unless it is made with pasteurized eggs and milk. Store-bought ice cream is safe.

Homemade mayonnaise ⚠️

Mayonnaise is made from vegetable oil, egg yolks (*see* Eggs), lemon juice or vinegar, and other seasonings.

CONCERNS: Since the eggs in homemade mayonnaise are not cooked, there is a possibility that they could contain a bacterium called *Salmonella* (*see Salmonella*). *Salmonella* can cause diarrhea, fever, and abdominal pain. It is most dangerous in people who have a weakened immune system. Women who are pregnant do not appear to be at an increased risk of getting *Salmonella*. However, one type of this bacterium can cross the placenta and cause miscarriage, stillbirth, and preterm labor.

THE BOTTOM LINE: You should avoid homemade mayonnaise unless it is made with pasteurized eggs. Store-bought mayonnaise is safe.

Honey ☑️

Honey is a sweet, thick liquid made by bees from flower nectar.

CONCERNS: Honey is sometimes contaminated with botulinum spores, which can cause botulism. Very young children should not eat honey because their digestive systems cannot prevent the botulinum spores from growing. An adult woman's digestive system will inhibit these spores from growing and will prevent botulism from occurring.

THE BOTTOM LINE: Honey is safe in pregnancy.

Horseback riding ⚠️ ∴

Horseback riding is the exercise of riding a horse, either English or western style.

CONCERNS: There are two concerns involving horseback riding. The first is the bouncing effect, and the second is the potential of falling. No scientific studies specifically examining the effects of bouncing during horseback riding on pregnancy could be found. Most physicians recommend that you abstain from any exercise (*see* Exercise) that has a high risk of falling during pregnancy. Falling and abdominal trauma have been associated with placental abruption (premature separation of the placenta), which can be very dangerous to both mother and child.

THE BOTTOM LINE: Horseback riding is probably safe in the first trimester. However, horseback riding puts you at risk for falling and abdominal trauma and should probably be avoided as your pregnancy progresses.

Hospital germs

Hospital germs are bacteria and viruses that are specifically found in hospitals and other health care facilities. Because there are many very sick people in hospitals, drug-resistant types of bacteria have evolved there.

CONCERNS: Because hospitals are known to have drug-resistant strains of bacteria, some women are cautious about delivering in the hospital and exposing their newborn babies to these bacteria. However, hospitals are extremely careful in controlling the spread of these drug-resistant bacteria. Most people on the labor and delivery units are healthy, and contact with drug-resistant bacteria in those units is extremely rare.

THE BOTTOM LINE: Hospitals do harbor drug-resistant strains of bacteria. However, these strains are most often found on units where there are very sick people, such as the intensive care units. If a strain of drug-resistant bacteria is found, the hospital does everything that it can to isolate these bacteria and prevent their spread to other units and patients. Avoid visiting very sick people while pregnant, and wash your hands carefully when coming into close contact with them.

Hot baths and hot showers

Hot baths and showers can be taken at home, at the health club, or at a spa. Home and public water heaters are generally set between 100°F/38°C and 110°F/43°C, with a maximum of 120°F/49°C, to help protect from bathtub scald or burn.

CONCERNS: Numerous studies have made an association between elevated temperatures and the increased incidence of neural tube defects and miscarriages. Hot baths appear to be dangerous if your core body temperature (CBT) rises to 102.5°F. Some researchers have suggested that if a pregnant woman's CBT becomes that high, she would feel uncomfortable and get out of the tub. Taking a hot shower does not usually result in an increased CBT.

THE BOTTOM LINE: Keeping bathwater below 100°F should be okay. If you don't have a thermometer handy, dip your elbow or forearm into the water. If the water is a comfortable temperature, it is probably safe. If your skin becomes red or you notice that you are sweating, the water is probably too hot.

Hot dogs

Hot dogs, a.k.a. frankfurters, are made of either pork or beef and are often topped with mustard, sauerkraut, beans, relish, cheese, and/or ketchup.

CONCERNS: A study in 2001 by the Food Safety and Inspection Service of the United States Department of Agriculture (FSIS/USDA) determined that many pregnant women were either not aware of the dangers of certain foods or did not handle these foods properly in the home. It is important to know that you are at risk for several foodborne illnesses that can be contracted through eating improperly prepared hot dogs during pregnancy.

Listeria (*see Listeria*) and *Campylobacter* (*see Campylobacter*) can contaminate hot dogs. Pregnant women are 20 times more likely to get listeriosis than other healthy adults. Infection with *Listeria* and *Campylobacter* can both cause preterm labor, miscarriage, and stillbirth. It is important to follow USDA recommendations on storage times and promptly refrigerate all hot dogs and deli meats. Make sure your refrigerator is set to 40°F/4.5°C or below. Do not use if the product freshness date has passed. Cooking these foods until steaming hot or using a meat thermometer (heat to 165°F/74°C) will ensure that all of the harmful bacteria are killed.

Hot dogs cured with nitrates and nitrites (*see Nitrates and nitrites*) have been associated with low birth weights and methemoglobinemia (a blood disorder resulting in low oxygen) in laboratory animals.

THE BOTTOM LINE: Careful cooking prior to eating will eliminate any harmful bacteria. Do not eat hot dogs unless they are steaming hot. Do not forget to clean up properly so you do not contaminate other foods with unwashed cutting boards (*see* Cutting boards) and knives. Consider nitrate-free hot dogs to reduce any risks to the baby.

Hot tubs

Hot tubs are large tubs filled with heated water. Most hot tubs are set between 100°F/38°C and 120°F/49°C. Many hot tubs also have jets of water. One popular brand of hot tub is the Jacuzzi®.

CONCERNS: Numerous studies have shown an association between elevated temperatures and the increased incidence of neural tube defects and miscarriages. Hot tubs appear to be dangerous if your core body temperature (CBT) rises to 102.5°F/39°C. Some researchers have suggested that if a pregnant woman's CBT becomes that high, she would feel uncomfortable and get out of the tub.

Hot tubs have also been used during labor for pain control and relaxation. One study has noted that women who used hot tubs during labor requested epidural analgesia less frequently due to less discomfort. The increased temperatures may be responsible for elevations in fetal heart rate, so if you use a hot tub during labor, the baby's heart rate should be checked intermittently. If the heart rate rises, you may be asked to get out of the tub.

Finally, some women have concerns over the risk of infections transmitted through hot tubs. To prevent this, most tubs are disinfected using chlorine (*see* Chlorine). A few studies have found that a group of byproducts of chlorine, trihalomethanes (THMs), can be found in water treated with chlorine and are associated with low birth weight and fetal birth defects, such as neural tube defects. THMs can be absorbed through the skin or lungs. It is unclear what levels are dangerous during pregnancy. Other studies have not found this association. Chlorine can also break down into chloroform, which may also cause harm during pregnancy. The Environmental Protection Agency has set up standards to monitor these levels and is continuing to do research on this issue.

THE BOTTOM LINE: It is probably best to avoid the use of hot tubs during pregnancy, especially in the first trimester, when the baby's organs are forming. If you are closely monitored, a properly cleaned and maintained hot tub appears to be safe during labor and useful for easing the pain of labor. Rinse off any chlorinated water after use.

Household cleaners

Household cleaners include a variety of commercially available products to clean the home. Common cleaners include bleach, ammonia, oven cleaners, and furniture polish.

CONCERNS: Many household cleaners are poisonous or harmful if ingested or with prolonged contact to the skin. Many contain volatile organic compounds, some of which are potentially carcinogenic (cancer causing). Not many of the common household cleaners have been tested in pregnancy, and they may pose health and environmental threats. No link has been seen between household cleaners and birth defects, and most are considered to be safe if used as directed. For now, use common sense with these cleaners. This includes wearing gloves and keeping the area well ventilated. If you are very concerned, try some of the more environmentally safe products, which are increasingly available.

THE BOTTOM LINE: Although household cleaners are probably safe in pregnancy, use precautions and limit your exposure when working with them. Never mix any chemicals, as the fumes are potentially dangerous.

Humidifiers

Humidifiers are machines that humidify the air by vaporizing water. They may create cold-water vapor or may have a heating unit to warm the water to make warm vapor.

CONCERNS: As with air conditioners and dehumidifiers (*see* Air conditioners; Dehumidifiers), there has been some publicity about the association of Legionnaire's disease outbreaks with humidifiers. Legionnaire's disease is caused by a bacterium called *legionellae*, which lives in warm-water environments like those found in air conditioners, plumbing systems, and humidifiers. It is estimated that 8,000 to 10,000 people contract Legionnaire's disease every year. However, it is often difficult to diagnose the disease accurately because symptoms can vary from person to person. Unless a doctor specifically suspects Legionnaire's, the appropriate tests are often not performed. The disease is most dangerous to those who have a weakened immune system due to cancer therapy, smoking, or organ transplant. Pregnancy does not appear to be an increased risk factor for getting this disease. While the U.S. Department of Labor's Occupational Safety and Health Administration has standards in place for work-related systems, it is unclear how many cases of Legionnaire's disease are acquired in private homes and what the optimal methods of prevention are. Proper maintenance of all plumbing systems, air-conditioning systems, and humidifiers should minimize your risk of contracting this disease.

Humidifiers are also great places for mold to grow. Some people are allergic to mold, so your humidifier should be properly cleaned and maintained. Follow the manufacturer's suggestions for proper maintenance.

Humidifier fever is a disease of unclear origin that occurs a few hours after exposure to a humidifier and is characterized by a flu-like illness that generally subsides within 24 hours. It is thought to be due to microorganisms (possibly mold or bacteria) that can grow inside the humidifier. Proper maintenance may prevent this from occurring.

THE BOTTOM LINE: A well-maintained humidifier is safe in pregnancy and may be beneficial for reducing the discomfort of dry skin and nasal passageways.

Humidity

Humidity describes how much moisture is in the air.

CONCERNS: Both low and high humidity have been associated with asthma (*see* Asthma) exacerbations. In conditions of high humidity, some allergens, such as molds, are able to grow at a faster rate. Low humidity has also been associated with dry skin and dry nasal passageways leading to bleeding inside the nose.

To control the humidity in your home, you can use either a humidifier (*see* Humidifiers) or a dehumidifier (*see* Dehumidifiers). The optimal humidity inside the home should be between 40 and 50 percent.

THE BOTTOM LINE: Both low and high humidity can cause discomfort during pregnancy. The optimal humidity in your home should be between 40 and 50 percent. Proper maintenance of humidifiers and dehumidifiers will ensure their safety.

Ibuprofen

Ibuprofen is a nonsteroidal anti-inflammatory drug (NSAID) that is used as a pain reliever (*see* Pain relievers) and anti-inflammatory, and as a fever reducer. Common brand names for ibuprofen include Advil®, Motrin®, and Nuprin®.

CONCERNS: Ibuprofen use during pregnancy has not been associated with any congenital birth defects, preterm labor, or low birth weight. However, its use has been associated with an increased risk of miscarriage in the first trimester, the premature closure of the ductus arteriosus (a part of the baby's heart) and oligohydramnios (low amniotic fluid level) when used in the third trimester. Thus, ibuprofen has been assigned a risk factor category of B in early pregnancy and a risk factor category of D in the third trimester (*see* Appendix 1). In addition, a recent review of over 36,000 women who took NSAIDs in the first trimester showed an association between NSAID use and birth defects, especially cardiac defects. This study showed that 7 percent of these women had a baby with at least one malformation. If future research confirms these findings, the U.S. Food and Drug Administration (FDA) may need to change the risk factor category of these medications.

THE BOTTOM LINE: Although ibuprofen currently has a risk factor category of B in the first two trimesters, it is recommended that you avoid this drug throughout pregnancy, but especially in the third trimester.

Ice cream, homemade *See* Homemade ice cream.

Immunizations ⚠️ ⠂⠂

Immunizations, a.k.a. vaccinations, are given to build immunity and prevent the development of a specific disease. Most immunizations are given during childhood, but some are given throughout adulthood.

CONCERNS: Since some immunizations are made from inactivated virus or part of a virus, many are not recommended during pregnancy due to concerns about birth defects and spreading the illness to the fetus. However, certain immunizations are suggested because the benefits outweigh the risks. The Centers for Disease Control and Prevention frequently updates these recommendations based on the safety of vaccinations given intentionally or inadvertently (before a woman knows she is pregnant) during pregnancy and in certain specific situations.

- *Contraindicated vaccines during pregnancy:* measles, mumps, rubella, yellow fever
- *Recommended during pregnancy:* influenza (*see* Flu vaccination) for all women in every trimester
- *Recommended on a case-by-case basis:* polio, rabies, hepatitis A, hepatitis B, pneumococcus, meningococcus, typhoid, anthrax, and tetanus

THE BOTTOM LINE: Your health care provider can discuss which immunizations are recommended during pregnancy.

Insect repellents ⚠️

Insect repellents are chemicals that are used to kill insects. The active chemical in the most effective insect repellents is diethyltoluamide, better known as DEET (*see* DEET). Insect repellents can be in the form of sprays and creams.

CONCERNS: Concern over the use of DEET increased after several reports of seizures in young children exposed to it. DEET is also known to be absorbed through the skin and can cross the placenta in animal studies. There is limited information about DEET use during pregnancy. However, in one known case, a child born to a woman who used DEET throughout her pregnancy had birth defects. Overall, DEET is considered to be safe for use during pregnancy and should be used, as the risks of

DEET use appear to be less than that of West Nile virus, which is transmitted by infected mosquitoes.

DEET preparations come in varying concentrations, generally ranging from 5 to 30 percent, although higher concentrations are available. The lower concentrations are active for shorter periods of time and may need to be reapplied after a couple of hours. Reapplication may be necessary after prolonged time spent outside or after swimming.

The Centers for Disease Control and Prevention (CDC) has the following recommendations for using insect repellents:

- Use enough repellent to cover exposed skin or clothing. Don't apply repellent to skin that is under clothing. Heavy application is not necessary to achieve protection.
- Do not apply repellent to cuts, wounds, or irritated skin. After returning indoors, wash treated skin with soap and water.
- Do not spray aerosol or pump products in enclosed areas.
- Do not spray aerosol or pump products directly on your face. Spray your hands and then rub them carefully over the face, avoiding eyes and mouth.

The Environmental Protection Agency and the CDC have been investigating new alternatives to DEET. Currently, the CDC endorses the use of picaridin repellents with 7 percent active ingredient and repellents with 30 percent oil of lemon eucalyptus (not for children under the age of three) as the active ingredient, which provide protection equal to a low-concentration DEET product. These products have not been extensively studied in pregnancy.

THE BOTTOM LINE: DEET is not contraindicated in pregnancy. Use as instructed, try to limit exposure time, and wash hands carefully after application.

Insecticides, home use
Insecticides are used to kill insects. Commonly used insecticides in the home are used to kill fleas, mosquitoes, ants, and cockroaches.

CONCERNS: Women exposed to household insecticides appear 1.5 times more likely to have a child with a birth defect. The most common defects noted were neural tube defects, facial defects, and limb defects.

The greatest risk appears to be associated with exposure during the first trimester and with prolonged exposure.

THE BOTTOM LINE: The safest thing to do is to avoid all insecticides throughout your pregnancy and especially during the first trimester. Early and prolonged exposure appears to lead to an increased risk of birth defects. If you must use these products, have someone else do the spraying, stay out of the room for the directed amount of time, wear gloves and a mask, and use in well-ventilated areas. If your skin is inadvertently exposed to insecticides or if they are ingested, call poison control.

Insecticides, outdoor use

Insecticides are used to kill insects to increase the yield of agricultural crops and to limit disease-spreading mosquitoes.

CONCERNS: Women living one-quarter mile from agricultural crops sprayed with insecticides appear 1.5 times more likely to have a baby with a birth defect. Insecticides have also been associated with attention deficit hyperactivity disorder.

THE BOTTOM LINE: Insecticides appear to be associated with an increased risk of birth defects. However, by limiting exposure, you can reduce much of the risk. Limiting exposure includes avoiding the area while spraying takes place, remaining outside the sprayed area for eight hours, and using adequate ventilation.

Iodine tablets

Iodine is a naturally occurring element that is necessary for a healthy thyroid gland and to properly metabolize fat. Iodine can be consumed from iodized salt, vegetables grown in iodine-rich soil (asparagus, garlic, lima beans, mushrooms, soybeans, spinach), kelp, and seafood. It is also found in dairy products from cows that are fed iodine-supplemented feed or use iodine-enriched salt licks. Most Americans get three times as much iodine in their diets as is needed, so deficiency is rare.

CONCERNS: Iodine deficiency has been associated with breast cancer, fetal hypothyroidism (low thyroid hormone), and weight gain. Some people have used iodine supplementation in an attempt to lose weight.

Toxicity to iodine tablets can occur. Iodine tablets are not recommended in pregnancy due to the risk of causing thyroid problems in the fetus.

THE BOTTOM LINE: A daily prenatal vitamin (*see* Multivitamins) will cover your iodine needs. Supplements should not be taken unless prescribed by a physician.

Iron

Iron is a mineral important in the production of new red blood cells. Adequate iron intake during pregnancy will help reduce the risk of the development of maternal anemia. Iron can be found in meat, fish, nuts, seeds, eggs, wheat germ, whole-grain products, and beans.

CONCERNS: All bottles of iron list a warning to keep out of the reach of children because iron toxicity can result from the ingestion of too much iron.

Many women develop anemia during pregnancy due to an increased blood volume. To counteract this, daily requirements are increased from 18 to 30 milligrams iron per day. Iron supplements may upset your stomach and contribute to constipation. Sometimes switching the brand or type of iron will make them more tolerable. Make sure to get adequate amounts of fiber in your diet to prevent constipation. Taking iron with vitamin C (*see* Vitamin C) or a Vitamin C–rich food, such as tomato juice, orange juice, or strawberries, will help with absorption of iron. Calcium (*see* Calcium) and some of the chemicals found in tea (*see* Camomile tea; Herb tea; Tea) and coffee (*see* Coffee) can make it more difficult to absorb iron.

THE BOTTOM LINE: Your iron requirements increase during pregnancy to 30 mg elemental iron per day. If you get enough iron in your diet and your prenatal vitamins, you may not need a supplement. If you have anemia related to iron deficiency or a multiple pregnancy (twins or more), your health care provider may recommend that you take an additional iron supplement.

Isotretinoin

Isotretinoin, sold under the brand name Accutane®, is a prescription drug used to treat severe acne. It is a synthetic form of Vitamin A (*see* Vitamin A).

CONCERNS: The manufacturer suggests that women use two forms of birth control for at least one month prior to beginning Accutane® and for one month after stopping the drug. This cautious approach is because isotretinoin is known to cause birth defects in 25 to 35 percent of women who take it during the first trimester of pregnancy. As a result, this drug has been assigned a pregnancy risk factor category of X, which means it should not be taken in pregnancy (*see* Appendix 1).

THE BOTTOM LINE: Isotretinoin increases your risk of miscarriage, birth defects, and fetal death. This drug should definitely be avoided. Further, you should wait at least one month after stopping isotretinoin before becoming pregnant. If you are pregnant and have been taking Accutane®, stop taking the medication immediately and call your health care provider.

Jacuzzi®

Jacuzzi® is a brand of hot tub (*see* Hot tubs).

Jasmine tea

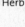

Jasmine tea is a tea made from an infusion of jasmine flowers (*see* Herb tea; Tea).

Juices

Juices are beverages made from fruits or vegetables, water, and sometimes sweeteners. Common examples include apple, carrot, and cranberry juice.

CONCERNS: Some women may need to limit the amount of juice that they drink if they are getting too many calories per day. Watch out for juices that are sweetened with artificial sweeteners (*see* Artificial sweeteners).

Other concerns center on the risks of drinking unpasteurized juices (*see* Unpasteurized juice) that could contain harmful bacteria, such as *Escherichia coli* or *Salmonella* (*see* Salmonella). The U.S. Food and Drug Administration requires unpasteurized juices to be labeled as such.

THE BOTTOM LINE: Pasteurized juice is safe in pregnancy. Be careful not to consume too many extra calories.

Keflex®

Keflex® is the brand name for the antibiotic cephalexin (*see* Antibiotics, oral; Cephalexin).

Kickboxing *See* Exercise.

Kwell®

Kwell® is the brand name for lindane (*see* Head lice).

Lansoprazole ⚠️

Lansoprazole, sold under the brand name Prevacid®, is an antacid (*see* Antacids). Lansoprazole is classified as a proton pump inhibitor (PPI). PPIs act to block acid secretion from cells in the stomach. Lansoprazole is used to treat gastroesophageal reflux disease (GERD).

CONCERNS: Lansoprazole has not been associated with any teratogenic (causing birth defects) effects. Lansoprazole has been assigned a risk factor category of B (*see* Appendix 1).

THE BOTTOM LINE: Lansoprazole appears to be safe in pregnancy at recommended doses.

Laxatives ⚠️

Laxatives are used in the treatment of constipation. Some women experience an increased rate of constipation during pregnancy that is due to increased hormonal levels that slow down the intestinal transit time, increased uterine size, changes in diet, prenatal vitamins, calcium supplements and antacids (*see* Antacids), and changes in exercise patterns (*see* Exercise). While increasing your fiber and water intake is considered to be the treatment of choice for constipation in pregnancy, occasionally you may be tempted to try a laxative.

Laxatives are categorized through their mechanism of action.

- *Cathartics* hold water in the intestines and thereby produce a watery stool. Examples of cathartic diuretics include Milk of Magnesia® (magnesium hydroxide) and Epsom salts (magnesium sulfate).

- *Stimulants* increase the movement of the intestines to cause a bowel movement. Examples of stimulants include Dulco-lax® (bisadocyl) and castor oil (*see* Castor oil).

- *Bulking agents* act to bulk up the stool to make having a bowel movement easier. Examples of bulking agents include Citrucel® (methylcellulose) and Metamucil® (psyllium).

- *Stool softeners* act to soften the stool. An example of a common stool softener is Colace® (*see* Docusate).

- Other agents act to retard the absorption of water from the intestine. An example of this type of laxative is mineral oil (*see* Mineral oil).

CONCERNS: The chronic use of laxatives is known to cause electrolyte imbalances and impaired absorption of certain vitamins. Some laxatives may contribute to dehydration, which may trigger preterm contractions.

Most laxatives are considered to be safe in pregnancy and have been assigned a risk factor category of B or C (*see* Appendix 1).

THE BOTTOM LINE: The best way to treat constipation related to pregnancy is by increasing your fiber (*see* Fiber) and water intake. There should be no need for a laxative unless these measures fail. If you are considering a laxative, consult with your OB/GYN first.

L-carnitine ⚠

L-carnitine is a nutrient needed to make energy from fat. L-carnitine can be produced by the body or obtained by eating dairy products and red meat. Medical conditions that appear to be helped by L-carnitine supplementation include anorexia, chronic fatigue syndrome, hypoglycemia, male infertility, and coronary artery disease.

CONCERNS: Since pregnancy is a state that requires increased energy, health care providers have proposed supplementation of women's diets with L-carnitine. Most available studies have been performed on pregnant pigs. A human study has noted that women who developed preeclampsia (hypertension, protein in the urine, and swelling) had higher levels of L-carnitine. Although this is an interesting finding, more needs to be known before any recommendation regarding L-carnitine use during pregnancy can be made.

Since L-carnitine is categorized as a food supplement, it is not regulated by the Food and Drug Administration. Thus, there is no guarantee of the strength, purity, or safety of this product. You should inform your health care provider if you are taking any nutritional supplements.

THE BOTTOM LINE: Although there appears to be no problem with L-carnitine and pregnancy, very few scientific studies regarding its use during pregnancy have been performed. In light of this and the fact that L-carnitine deficiency is rare (even in strict vegetarians), it is probably safest to avoid this supplement during pregnancy until more is known about any potential effects.

Lead ⊘

Lead is a metal that naturally occurs in our environment. Most exposure to lead during pregnancy is through contaminated drinking water and soil, occupational exposure, and lead-based paint.

CONCERNS: It is now known that lead can cross the human placenta. Exposure to high levels of lead has been associated with spontaneous abortion, preterm labor, and premature rupture of membranes. Lead has never been linked to any major congenital abnormalities, but some studies have found a variety of minor malformations associated with high lead levels. Prenatal exposure to lead has also been associated with lower mental development scores in infants. However, these differences were noted to disappear after 24 months of age, leading researchers to conclude that the children either recovered from lead exposure or that the later tests could not pick up any deficts. In either event, it appears that postnatal exposure to lead has more significant effects on children than exposure during the prenatal period.

Studies using laboratory rats have concluded that lead in their drinking water may be responsible for the development of chronic diseases, such as asthma (*see* Asthma), cancer, and allergies.

THE BOTTOM LINE: Lead is suspected to be a teratogen (cause of birth defects), and unnecessary exposure during pregnancy should be avoided. Consider having your drinking water tested or use a filter. If you have lead pipes, running your water for several minutes prior to use in the morning will help decrease the amounts of lead consumed. If you are planning on doing any construction (*see* Building materials; Lead paint), have your walls tested for lead prior to tearing them down or sanding them so that appropriate precautions can be taken. If you have any occupational exposure to lead, you should have your levels monitored throughout the pregnancy.

Lead paint   🚫

Some paints, especially those used prior to 1950, contain lead. Household paints today do not contain lead, but use latex or oil.

CONCERNS: Exposure to lead during pregnancy can occur through contact with lead-based paint or through inhalation of dust particles from torn-down or sanded walls previously painted with lead-based paint. Lead has never been linked to any major congenital abnormalities, but some studies have found a variety of minor malformations associated with high lead levels. Prenatal exposure to lead has been associated with lower mental development scores in infants. However, these differences were noted to disappear after 24 months of age, leading researchers to conclude that the children either recovered from lead exposure or that the later tests could not pick up any deficits. In either event, it appears that postnatal exposure to lead has more significant effects on children than exposure during the prenatal period.

Studies using laboratory rats have concluded that lead in their drinking water may be responsible for the development of chronic diseases, such as asthma (*see* Asthma), cancer, and allergies.

THE BOTTOM LINE: Lead is suspected to be a teratogen (cause of birth defects), and unnecessary exposure during pregnancy should be avoided. If you are planning on doing any construction (*see* Building materials; Lead), have your walls tested for lead prior to tearing them down or sanding them so that appropriate precautions can be taken. If the house was built prior to 1950, it is likely that there will be lead paint (*see* Lead paint). If there is any sanding or demolition, consider wearing a mask or moving to a different location during the renovation.

Lecithin

Lecithin is a fat categorized as a phospholipid that is found in cell membranes. Lecithin is considered to be an essential nutrient and is found in eggs and meats. Currently there is no known recommended daily allowance for lecithin. Lecithin may play a role in keeping the cardiovascular system and liver healthy and in reproduction. Commercial lecithin supplements may be purchased in granular or capsule form.

CONCERNS: People may have reduced amounts of lecithin in their diets due to decreased fat intake. A large component in lecithin is choline. Adequate intake of choline during pregnancy has been associated with a decreased incidence of neural tube defects.

Because lecithin supplements are categorized as food supplements, they are not regulated by the U.S. Food and Drug Administration. Thus, there is no guarantee of the strength, purity, or safety of these products. You should inform your health care provider if you are taking any nutritional supplements.

THE BOTTOM LINE: Due to the fact that there are no clear recommended amounts for lecithin intake, caution should be used until further studies demonstrate its safety in pregnancy. If you were on a low-fat diet prior to pregnancy, consider increasing your fat intake to insure adequate consumption of lecithin.

Librium®

Librium® is a brand name for chlordiazepoxide (*see* Psychiatric medications).

Linoleic acid *See* Conjugated linoleic acid.

Liquor *See* Alcoholic beverages.

Listeria

Listeria monocytogenes is a bacterium that can contaminate unpasteurized milk, soft cheese (*see* Cheese), deli meats (*see* Deli meats, cooked and uncooked; Cured meat), refrigerated patés and meat spreads, and smoked fish (*see* Smoked fish). Infection with *Listeria* can cause listeriosis, a flu-like illness characterized by fever, chills, and muscle aches. The Centers for Disease Control and Prevention (CDC) estimates that approximately 2,500 people become seriously ill with listeriosis per year.

CONCERNS: Pregnant women are 20 times more likely to get listeriosis than other healthy adults. Infection during pregnancy may lead to preterm labor and even stillbirth.

Listeria can contaminate unpasteurized milk, soft cheese, deli meats, refrigerated patés and meat spreads, and smoked fish despite proper storage and refrigeration. The risk of contamination can be decreased, but not prevented, by keeping your refrigerator at 40°F/4.5°C or below; keeping your refrigerator clean; avoiding cross-contamination from countertops, cutting boards (*see* Cutting boards), and utensils; and not leaving foods unrefrigerated for more than two hours. Deli meats should be well cooked prior to eating. Cooking soft cheese to boiling/bubbling will ensure your safety.

THE BOTTOM LINE: Currently, the CDC has recommended that pregnant women avoid soft cheese such as brie (*see* Brie), camembert (*see* Camembert), feta (*see* Feta), blue-veined cheeses (*see* Blue-veined cheese), and Mexican-style cheeses (*see* Mexican-style cheese) and unpasteurized milk. It is recommended that all deli meats be heated until steaming during pregnancy.

Lithium

Lithium is a mood stabilizer used in the treatment of bipolar disorder (*see* Psychiatric medications).

Litter boxes

Litter boxes contain clay or paper particles and are used as places where cats urinate and defecate (*see* Cats).

CONCERNS: *Toxoplasmosis gondii* (*see* Toxoplasmosis) is a parasite that can be transmitted through the feces of cats, *Toxoplasmosis* infection can cause fetal death, preterm labor, and some kinds of birth defects. However, *Toxoplasmosis* is a common childhood infection. Many people are immune to it, and a quick blood test from your health care provider will reveal whether you are immune. If you are immune, there is no need to worry. If you are susceptible, or not immune, you have several options. You can test your cat, keep it indoors, have someone else change the litter pan, or wash your hands very carefully after emptying the litter pan.

THE BOTTOM LINE: Wash hands carefully after changing the cat litter, or, better yet, have someone else do this chore.

Loratadine

Loratadine is an antihistamine (*see* Allergy medications; Antihistamines). A brand name for this drug is Claritin®.

CONCERNS: Loratadine has been assigned a risk factor category of B (*see* Appendix 1).

THE BOTTOM LINE: Loratadine is safe to take during pregnancy.

Lubricants

Lubricants are often used for comfort during sexual intercourse and during pelvic examinations in your provider's office. Most are water-based like K-Y Jelly®, while some are petroleum-based like Vaseline.

CONCERNS: There are some reports that lubricants used while trying to conceive may result in decreased sperm counts. Petroleum-based lubricants have also been associated with changes in vaginal flora leading to vaginal infections; they can also degrade latex condoms. However, if you are already pregnant and your cervix is closed, it is unlikely that any of the lubricant will enter the uterine cavity.

THE BOTTOM LINE: Water-based lubricants are completely safe during pregnancy.

Lutein

Lutein is a chemical that is related to the carotenoids and is classified as an antioxidant. It may help correct damage to cells caused by free radicals, and some studies suggest that it may be useful in the protection of eyesight. Lutein can be found in spinach, peas, collard greens, and kale.

CONCERNS: Since lutein supplements are categorized as a food supplement, they are not regulated by the U.S. Food and Drug Administration. Thus, there is no guarantee of the strength, purity, or safety of these products. You should inform your health care provider if you are taking any nutritional supplements.

THE BOTTOM LINE: Although lutein appears to be beneficial and there have been no reports of pregnancy-related problems, there are no known safe levels of lutein during pregnancy.

Lycopene

Lycopene is a chemical classified as an antioxidant that may help correct damage to cells caused by free radicals. Some people think that lycopene may reduce the risks of certain cancers, reduce the effects of sun damage, and improve asthma and coronary artery disease. Lycopene can be found in tomatoes and tomato-based products.

CONCERNS: A small study showed an association between lycopene supplementation and a decreased risk of developing preeclampsia (hypertension, protein in the urine, and swelling) and intrauterine growth restriction (low birth weight).

Because lycopene supplements are categorized as food supplements, they are not regulated by the U.S. Food and Drug Administration. Thus, there is no guarantee of the strength, purity, or safety of these products. You should inform your health care provider if you are taking any nutritional supplements.

THE BOTTOM LINE: Although lycopene appears to be beneficial and there have been no reports of pregnancy-related problems, there are no known safe levels of lycopene during pregnancy.

Lyme disease

Lyme disease is caused by a parasite called *Borrelia burgdorferi*, which is transmitted to humans through ticks. The initial stage of the disease generally appears as a rash called a target lesion that looks like a bull's-eye. If untreated at this stage, the disease can progress and cause a variety of conditions, including flu-like illness, headache, chronic neurological conditions, arthritis, and cardiac disease.

CONCERNS: It is known that the parasite can cross the placenta and cause disease in the fetus. Some reports have shown an association between Lyme disease during pregnancy and miscarriage, fetal infection, fetal abnormalities, and fetal death. However, the evidence does not clearly support a strong association between Lyme disease during pregnancy and adverse pregnancy outcomes.

Insecticides containing DEET (*see* DEET) can protect you from ticks, which transmit Lyme disease. Concern over the use of DEET increased after several reports of seizures in young children exposed to DEET. DEET is also known to be absorbed through the skin and can cross the placenta in animal studies. There is limited information about DEET use during pregnancy. Overall, DEET is considered to be safe for use during pregnancy.

THE BOTTOM LINE: Lyme disease is potentially dangerous during pregnancy. If you live in an area affected by Lyme disease, consider reducing your risk by dressing appropriately, checking for ticks after returning inside, and using an insect repellent containing DEET. DEET is not contraindicated in pregnancy. Use as instructed, try to limit exposure, and wash hands carefully after application. Notify your health care provider if you suspect that you have been infected with Lyme disease, as early treatment with antibiotics can reduce the severity of disease.

Maalox®

Maalox® is a brand name for an antacid (*see* Antacids).

Macrodantin®

Macrodantin® is the brand name for the antibiotic nitrofurantoin (*see* Antibiotics, oral; Nitrofurantoin).

Magnesium

Magnesium is an element that is needed for the repair of damaged tissue, for building bones and teeth, and to make certain enzymes function properly. Magnesium is found in green leafy vegetables, whole grains, nuts, meats, and milk. Magnesium can also be purchased as a nutritional supplement. Magnesium is a component of many prenatal vitamins. The Recommended Daily Allowance for magnesium during pregnancy is 450 milligrams.

CONCERNS: Women with poor diets are more likely to be deficient in magnesium. Magnesium supplementation during pregnancy has been investigated and has been associated with a reduction in preterm labor and preeclampsia (hypertension, protein in the urine, and swelling) and increased birth weight. However, a recent review failed to confirm any differences between supplementation with magnesium and a placebo.

THE BOTTOM LINE: There is not enough evidence to show that magnesium supplementation in pregnancy has any beneficial or deleterious effect.

Malathion

Malathion is an insect repellent (*see* Insecticides), typically used in agriculture and in the home.

CONCERNS: Several case reports associate exposure of children to malathion with gastrointestinal and immunological problems. Frogs and turtles exposed to malathion also seem to have increased birth defects. There are no data evaluating the human teratogenic (cause of birth defects) effects of malathion.

THE BOTTOM LINE: Not much information is available on the effects of malathion exposure during pregnancy. It seems reasonable to avoid this and all insecticides whenever possible.

Manicures

Manicures are treatments performed on the hands and fingernails that can include shaping, cleaning, and polishing (*see* Acrylic nails; Nail polish).

CONCERNS: Because most manicurists find it necessary to wear face masks to avoid breathing in fumes, many pregnant women have concerns about having manicures and about visiting salons where manicures are performed. It is also known that some chemicals can be absorbed into the natural nail itself.

Recent reports from the U.S. Food and Drug Administration indicate that the chemicals used in nail polish and in nail polish removers are potentially dangerous and can cause skin irritation and rashes. Chemicals that are particularly dangerous include methyl methacrylate (MMA), acetonitrile, and formaldehyde. Some manicurists have begun using products that appear to be safer, in that they do not contain any of the listed harsh chemicals.

There have been some reports about an increased incidence of infections of the nail bed following cuticle treatments. This risk does not seem to be increased during pregnancy.

THE BOTTOM LINE: No studies deal specifically with manicures and pregnancy, and no available case reports suggest an association with bad pregnancy outcomes. If you are worried about any potential effects, avoid the treatment outright while pregnant. Make every effort to limit potential effects by waiting until after the first trimester, when there is less risk to the development of the baby's organs; go to a well-ventilated salon, visit earlier in the day when there are less fumes, consider wearing a mask, and avoid getting chemicals on your skin. Nail treatments without nail polish are safe.

Marijuana ⚠️

Marijuana, or cannabis, is a plant that can be dried and then smoked. Some people who smoke marijuana report that it has a calming effect and can increase appetite. Marijuana is considered to be a drug of abuse (see Drugs of abuse) and is illegal in this country. Marijuana has been found to help with morning sickness and nausea related to cancer therapy, and to increase appetite. There is a movement to allow its legal use as a medication, and several states have already legalized its use for medical therapy.

CONCERNS: Smoking marijuana prior to pregnancy has been associated with decreased male and female fertility.

Several studies have associated marijuana use during pregnancy with low birth weight and neurological delays; others have not seen this association. One large retrospective study that was able to show an association between low birth weight and marijuana use found that when patients who also used tobacco were eliminated from the study results, an association was no longer seen. Occasional use of marijuana has not been associated with any birth defects.

THE BOTTOM LINE: It is still unclear whether occasional marijuana use is safe in pregnancy. Until we learn more about its effects during pregnancy, and until it is legal in the United States, its use during pregnancy cannot be recommended.

Massage ☑️

Massage is the kneading or rubbing of parts of the body to promote relaxation and decrease muscle soreness.

CONCERNS: A recent study found that pregnant women who received a massage two times per week for five weeks had better sleep patterns, lower anxiety levels, less back pain, and lower levels of stress hormones. Other studies have shown an association between prenatal massage and decreased preterm labor and neonatal problems. Massage is also known to reduce the pain during labor. The concern over foot massage during pregnancy centers on the risk of initiating preterm labor as a result of stimulation of certain "touch points" on the foot. However, I could find no scientific studies that examined this possibility. One study did demonstrate that foot massage correlated with an increase in fetal movements at midgestation (around 20 weeks).

THE BOTTOM LINE: Massage appears to be safe and beneficial during pregnancy. Look for a referral from the American Massage Therapy Association, and ask if the practitioner has specific experience with prenatal massage.

Measles

Measles, also known as rubeola, is a disease caused by a virus. Most children in the United States are vaccinated against measles, and as a result, the incidence of this disease has become very low.

CONCERNS: Pregnant women are not more likely to get the measles, but they are at risk for more serious complications and death due to developing pneumonia. Measles can also affect the baby, causing preterm labor, postnatal measles, and fetal death. There does not appear to be an increased risk of congenital defects. Due to these facts, many women who seek preconception counseling (counseling prior to becoming pregnant) will be offered a measles vaccine if they are found to be nonimmune. If you discover that you do not have immunity during your pregnancy, you will be offered vaccination after the delivery of your baby.

THE BOTTOM LINE: Most women are immune to the measles as a result of routine childhood vaccinations. Your health care provider will check for this immunity by doing a blood test prior to pregnancy or at your first prenatal visit. If you are not immune, you should be careful to avoid contact with anyone known to have the measles.

Melatonin ⚠

Melatonin is a hormone produced by the brain and is known to be at its highest levels during sleep. Melatonin is commonly used to treat insomnia and to reduce jet lag. It can be purchased in a tablet or capsule form. The melatonin products being sold are synthetic or made from animal pineal glands.

CONCERNS: The ideal doses of melatonin during pregnancy are currently not known.

Because melatonin is categorized as a food supplement, it is not regulated by the U.S. Food and Drug Administration. Thus, there is no guarantee of the strength, purity, or safety of this product. You should inform your health care provider if you are taking any nutritional supplements.

THE BOTTOM LINE: Even if you have some difficulty sleeping during your pregnancy, the use of melatonin has not been adequately studied and is therefore not recommended.

Mercury ⚠

Mercury is a metal that occurs naturally in our environment and is also a by-product of some industrial processes. Mercury can be ingested via inhalation, by eating contaminated foods, or through direct skin contact.

CONCERNS: Exposure to mercury causes both acute and chronic toxicity, including upper respiratory disease, neurological disease, and kidney disease. Appropriate precautions should be taken when working with mercury.

Some people have concerns over dental fillings made with mercury (amalgam fillings). However, the American Dental Association has researched this topic and has failed to detect any significant problems related to the mercury in the fillings. Mercury can be converted to methylmercury (see Methylmercury) by certain bacteria and can accumulate in certain species of fish (see Fish; Tuna). Finally, some providers have recommended avoiding influenza vaccines (see Flu vaccination) due to their mercury content. Currently, the Centers for Disease Control and Prevention recommends that all pregnant women receive the flu vaccine.

The effect of mercury on pregnancy has not been adequately studied. Experiments on laboratory animals showed an association with intrauterine growth restriction (low birth weight), birth defects, and fetal death.

THE BOTTOM LINE: Mercury is a potentially harmful material. If you have occupational exposure to mercury, please let your employer know that you are pregnant, check the Occupational Safety and Health Administration (OSHA) guidelines, and take the appropriate precautions.

Meringue

Meringue is a combination of stiffly beaten egg whites (*see* Eggs) and sugar. It often tops pies and desserts. After meringue is added to the desserts, they are generally baked at low temperatures.

CONCERNS: Raw and undercooked eggs could contain a bacterium called *Salmonella* (*see Salmonella*). *Salmonella* can cause diarrhea, fever, and abdominal pain. It is most dangerous in people who have a weakened immune system. Women who are pregnant do not appear to be at an increased risk of getting *Salmonella*. However, one type of this bacterium can cross the placenta and cause miscarriage, stillbirth, and preterm labor. If the meringue is cooked until hard, it is unlikely to contain any live *Salmonella*. However, if the meringue is soft, it is possible that it is contaminated with *Salmonella*.

THE BOTTOM LINE: Meringues that are baked until hard are safe. Although *Salmonella* is destroyed at 165°F/74°C, the internal temperature of a soft meringue may not be that high. Therefore, avoid soft meringues unless they are cooked at 135°F/57°C for 15 minutes or made with pasteurized eggs. Proper cleanup when cooking with eggs will help prevent cross-contamination.

Methylmercury

Mercury (*see* Mercury) is a metal that occurs naturally in our environment and is also a by-product of some industrial processes. Certain bacteria can convert naturally occurring and man-made mercury to methylmercury. Methylmercury can accumulate in the fatty tissue of certain fish (*see* Fish). Certain large predatory fish, such as shark, tuna, and swordfish, have the highest amount of methylmercury in their fat cells because they eat a lot of smaller fish.

CONCERNS: The U.S. Food and Drug Administration (FDA) has voiced concern over the methylmercury levels in many commonly consumed fish. When consumed in high doses, methylmercury is known to be harmful to a baby's developing neurologic system. The FDA has recommended safe amounts of different varieties of fish for pregnant women and young children. Keep in mind that these recommendations may change with the health of our ecosystems. Tuna (*see* Tuna), shark, swordfish, king mackerel, and tile fish (a.k.a. golden or white snapper) are known to contain high levels of this pollutant. The FDA recommends only two 6-ounce servings of these fish per week during pregnancy.

THE BOTTOM LINE: Consumption of large amounts of methylmercury may be dangerous for everyone, but especially during pregnancy and in early childhood. Follow the FDA guidelines to ensure that you are not consuming dangerous amounts of methylmercury.

Metrogel®

Metrogel® is the brand name for metronidazole (*see* Metronidazole; Antibiotics, topical).

Metronidazole

Metronidazole is an antibiotic commonly used for the treatment of bacterial vaginitis (*see* Bacterial vaginitis) and trichomoniasis (*see* Trichomoniasis; Parasites). A common brand name is Flagyl®.

CONCERNS: Metronidazole has a risk factor category of B (*see* Appendix 1). Despite this rating, the American College of Obstetrics and Gynecology recommends avoiding this antibiotic during the first trimester due to an association with facial abnormalities and childhood cancer.

THE BOTTOM LINE: Metronidazole is safe during pregnancy after the first trimester. It is important not to drink any alcoholic beverages while using metronidazole, as it can cause interactions that can damage the liver.

Mexican-style cheese

Common Mexican-style cheeses include queso blanco, queso fresco, queso de hoja, queso de crema, and asadero. They are all considered to be soft cheeses.

CONCERNS: Several outbreaks of *Listeria monocytogenes* (*see Listeria*) have been associated with the ingestion of queso fresco and cojita in California. These cheeses were homemade and sold door to door. Contamination of soft cheese with harmful bacteria such as *Listeria* can occur. This bacterium can cause preterm labor and stillbirth. The Centers for Disease Control and Prevention (CDC) recommends avoiding all soft cheese, including Mexican-style cheese, during pregnancy. The high sugar and moisture content of soft cheese is favorable for bacterial growth. The risk of contamination can be decreased, but not prevented, by keeping your refrigerator at 40°F/4.5°C or below; keeping your refrigerator clean; avoiding cross-contamination from countertops, cutting boards (*see* Cutting boards), and utensils; and not leaving foods unrefrigerated for more than two hours.

THE BOTTOM LINE: The CDC recommends avoiding Mexican-style cheese during pregnancy. Cooking the cheese until boiling/bubbling will eliminate any harmful bacteria.

Miconazole

Miconazole is the antifungal found in Monistat® (*see* Antifungal medications, oral and topical).

CONCERNS: Miconazole has been assigned a risk factor category of C (see Appendix 1). There have been no adverse pregnancy outcomes associated with topical miconazole.

THE BOTTOM LINE: Miconazole is considered to be safe in pregnancy.

Microwaves

Microwaves are a form of electromagnetic radiation with a long wavelength. Electromagnetic radiation produces electromagnetic fields (EMFs) (*see* Electric and magnetic fields). Direct exposure to microwaves affects cells by raising their temperatures.

CONCERNS: Some case reports suggest an association between EMFs and miscarriage, low birth weight, and congenital defects. No scientific studies have been able to show a clear association between EMFs and pregnancy complications. One study involving the exposure of pregnant rats to microwaves failed to show any adverse effects in pregnancy.

THE BOTTOM LINE: There is no scientific evidence that the routine use of microwave ovens causes any harm to a pregnancy.

Mineral oil ⚠

Mineral oil is a type of oil that can be used as a laxative (*see* Laxatives).

CONCERNS: The use of mineral oil as a laxative has been shown to interfere with the absorption of several nutrients and minerals. Mineral oil has been assigned a risk factor category of C (*see* Appendix 1).

THE BOTTOM LINE: Mineral oil is not recommended as a laxative during pregnancy. Constipation is best treated by increasing the amount of fiber and water in your diet.

Monistat® ✅

Monistat® is a brand name for miconazole (*see* Antifungal medications, oral and topical; Miconazole).

Motrin® ⚠ ∴

Motrin® is a brand name for ibuprofen (*see* Ibuprofen; Pain relievers).

Mousse ⚠

Mousse is a rich and airy dish that can either be sweet or savory. Dessert mousse is often made from fruit or chocolate, cream, and egg whites (*see* Eggs). Savory mousse is often made from meat, vegetables, cheese, and egg whites and then cooked over a double boiler. Mousse may sometimes contain wine (*see* Alcoholic beverages).

CONCERNS: Raw and undercooked eggs could contain a bacterium called *Salmonella* (*see* Salmonella). *Salmonella* can cause diarrhea, fever, and abdominal pain. It is most dangerous in people who have a weakened immune system. Women who are pregnant do not appear to be at an increased risk of getting *Salmonella*. However, one type of this bacterium can cross the placenta and cause miscarriage, stillbirth, and preterm labor. *Salmonella* is destroyed by cooking foods to 165°F/74°C.

Undercooked meat may be contaminated with *Listeria* (*see* Listeria) or *Campylobacter* (*see* Campylobacter). Pregnant women are 20 times more likely to get listeriosis than other healthy adults. Infected pregnant women may have symptoms similar to the flu, such as fever and muscle aches, and infection may lead to preterm labor and even stillbirth. Both *Listeria* and *Campylobacter* can cause preterm labor and stillbirth.

THE BOTTOM LINE: Mousse contains undercooked eggs, which can be contaminated with *Salmonella*. Avoid raw eggs during pregnancy or use pasteurized eggs. Careful cleaning of cutting boards (*see* Cutting boards) and utensils will help to prevent cross-contamination. When cooked over a double boiler, some meats may be undercooked and can become contaminated with *Listeria* and *Campylobacter*. Foods that contain alcohol should be avoided during pregnancy, unless the alcohol is burned off during the cooking process.

Mozzarella

Mozzarella (*see* Cheese) is an Italian-style cheese made by dipping the cheese curd into hot whey and then stretching and kneading it to the desired consistency. It can be made from the milk of water buffaloes or cows, or a combination of the two. Commercially processed or regular mozzarella is considered to be semisoft. Fresh mozzarella is considered to be a soft cheese.

CONCERNS: Since mozzarella can be made from raw (unpasteurized) milk, caution should be used during pregnancy (*see* Unpasteurized cheese). All cheese made in the United States is made only from pasteurized milk. The U.S. Food and Drug Administration allows the importation of raw-milk cheese into the United States only if the cheese is aged 60 days or more. The harmful bacteria die as a result of the aging process. Young cheese aged less than 60 days made from unpasteurized milk is not allowed into the country.

Even if the cheese you are eating is made from pasteurized milk, contamination of soft cheese with harmful bacteria such as *Listeria monocy-togenes* (*see* Listeria) can occur. This bacterium can cause preterm labor and stillbirth during pregnancy. The Centers for Disease Control and Prevention (CDC) recommends avoiding all soft cheese, including mozzarella, during pregnancy. The high sugar and moisture content of soft cheese is favorable for bacterial growth. The risk of contamination can be decreased, but not prevented, by keeping your refrigerator at 40°F/4.5°C or below; keeping your refrigerator clean; avoiding cross-contamination from countertops, cutting boards (*see* Cutting boards), and utensils; and not leaving cheese unrefrigerated for more than two hours.

THE BOTTOM LINE: Regular mozzarella made in the United States is safe. However, fresh mozzarella may become contaminated with *Listeria* and should be avoided during pregnancy unless cooked until boiling/bubbling. The importation of young cheese made with raw milk is prohibited, but use caution when in another country.

MSG

MSG, or monosodium glutamate, is a food additive (*see* Food additives). It is added to many foods as a flavor enhancer.

CONCERNS: Some people, whether pregnant or not, develop adverse reactions to MSG. These reactions include headache, nausea, vomiting, and sleep disturbances. Due to these reactions, MSG-containing foods must be labeled. If you are sensitive to MSG, make sure to ask if it is used when dining out.

The U.S. Food and Drug Administration has tested MSG and concluded that it is generally recognized as safe (GRAS). There have been mixed reports about MSG's capability of crossing the placenta into the fetal bloodstream. Studies in mice have shown that when ingested at high doses, it can cross the placenta and cause effects on the fetal brain. In a study of human pregnancy, the placenta did not allow MSG to cross into the baby's bloodstream.

THE BOTTOM LINE: MSG consumption appears to be safe during pregnancy. If you have any side effects from this food additive, remember to ask the chef not to use it. Careful label reading will allow you to identify foods that contain this product.

MSM

MSM, or methylsulfonylmethane, is a naturally occurring sulfur compound. It is found in fresh fruits and vegetables and in human cells. It is taken to relieve acne, to decrease inflammation, and to improve the quality of hair and nails. It can be purchased in the form of flakes, crystals, powders, tablets, lotions, and gels.

CONCERNS: Since MSM supplements are categorized as a food supplement, they are not regulated by the U.S. Food and Drug Administration. Thus, there is no guarantee of the strength, purity, or safety of these products. You should inform your health care provider if you are taking any nutritional supplements.

THE BOTTOM LINE: Not enough information is known about the effects of MSM during pregnancy. In light of this, it is recommended that you avoid this supplement.

Multivitamins

Multivitamins are preparations that contain an array of different vitamins and nutrients. Prenatal vitamins generally contain more of certain vitamins needed during pregnancy and can be purchased either over the counter or with a prescription. Pregnant women are routinely advised to take one a day prior to conceiving through pregnancy and the postpartum period.

CONCERNS: Proper nutrition and adequate intake of vitamins has been associated with increased health and a decreased risk of having a baby with a birth defect. For example, it is well known that folic acid (*see* Folic acid) supplementation can decrease the risk of having a child with a neural tube defect. Recent studies have demonstrated an association between multivitamin use during pregnancy and a reduction in certain types of childhood cancers in children and a reduction of AIDS symptoms in HIV-positive women.

Some women complain that taking a prenatal multivitamin during pregnancy causes them to feel nauseous. If this is the case, you can try a different formulation or try taking it at night prior to sleep.

THE BOTTOM LINE: Most health care providers recommend one prenatal multivitamin a day. It is not recommended that you take more than one a day, as certain vitamins may be toxic in high amounts.

Mushrooms ✓

Mushrooms are a fungus that comes in many varieties, shapes, colors, and flavors. Mushrooms can be cooked or eaten raw.

CONCERNS: Commercially available mushrooms are safe, but since there are many poisonous wild mushrooms, use care if not purchasing them in a food market. Some health care providers use mushrooms medicinally.

THE BOTTOM LINE: Commercially available mushrooms are safe to eat during pregnancy. The safety of medicinal mushroom use has not yet been established.

Mylanta® ✓

Mylanta® is a brand name for an antacid (*see* Antacids).

Mylicon® ✓

Mylicon® is a brand name for simethicone (*see* Simethicone).

Nail polish ✓

Nail polish is a clear or colored lacquer that can be applied to the finger-nails or toenails (*see* Manicures).

CONCERNS: Recent reports from the U.S. Food and Drug Administration indicate that the chemicals used in nail polish and in nail polish re-movers are potentially dangerous and can cause skin irritation and rashes. Other studies have shown that chemicals can be absorbed through the natural nail bed. Chemicals that are particularly dangerous include methyl methacrylate (MMA), acetonitrile, and formaldehyde. Some manicurists have begun using products that appear to be safer, in that they do not contain any of the listed harsh chemicals.

No scientific literature examining the effects of nail polish use during human pregnancy was found.

THE BOTTOM LINE: Some of the chemicals in nail polish have been as-sociated with skin conditions and birth defects. However, it is unclear if moderate use of these products on the nails will cause any pregnancy complications. If you opt to polish your nails, avoid MMA, acetonitrile, and formaldehyde; avoid getting polish on your skin; and use in a well-ventilated area.

Naphazoline ✓

Naphazoline is an antihistamine (*see* Allergy medications; Antihista-mines). A brand name for this drug is Allerest®.

CONCERNS: Naphazoline has been assigned a risk factor category of C (*see* Appendix 1).

THE BOTTOM LINE: Naphazoline is safe to take during pregnancy.

Naproxen

Naproxen is a nonsteroidal anti-inflammatory drug (NSAID) used in the treatment of pain (*see* Pain relievers) and inflammation, and as a fever reducer. A common brand name is Aleve®.

CONCERNS: Naproxen has been assigned a risk factor category of B in the first two trimesters and a risk factor category of D in the third trimester (*see* Appendix 1). A recent review of over 36,000 women who took NSAIDs in the first trimester showed an association between NSAID use and birth defects, especially cardiac defects. This study showed that 7 percent of these women had a baby with at least one malformation. If future research confirms these findings, the U.S. Food and Drug Administration (FDA) may need to change the risk factor category of these medications.

THE BOTTOM LINE: Although naproxen has a risk factor category of B in the first two trimesters, in light of recent studies, it is recommended that you avoid this drug throughout pregnancy, but especially in the third trimester.

Nasacort®

Nasacort® is a brand name of triamcinolone acetonide (*see* Triamcinolone acetonide; Allergy medications).

Nasal sprays

Nasal sprays are used in the nasal passages to reduce stuffiness and congestion. Up to 30 percent of pregnant women experience rhinitis (inflammation of the mucous membranes lining the nose) and stuffiness. Nasal sprays can contain several active ingredients, including saline, decongestants, and steroids.

CONCERNS: Because different nasal sprays vary in their ingredients, you need to read the labels carefully. Most medications can be absorbed through the nasal mucosa. However, the amount of drug absorbed is usually smaller when compared to oral medications. Saline nasal sprays are completely safe and can help with nasal congestion. Nasal sprays with decongestants (*see* Decongestants; Cough and cold suppressants) are considered to be safe as well, but may cause a rebound effect (worsening stuffiness after prolonged use), so their use should be limited. Doctor-prescribed corticosteroids (prescribed to decrease inflammation) are also considered to be safe in pregnancy and generally have been assigned a risk factor category of C (*see* Appendix 1).

THE BOTTOM LINE: Most nasal sprays are safe in pregnancy. However, due to a rebound effect seen in many sprays, their use should be limited.

Nexium®

Nexium® is a brand name for esomeprazole (*see* Esomeprazole; Antacids).

Niacin

Niacin, or Vitamin B_3, is a water-soluble B complex vitamin that is required for metabolism of lipids. The recommended daily allowance (RDA) during pregnancy is 17 milligrams. Niacin is found in meat, poultry, fish, dairy products, leafy green vegetables, legumes, and prenatal vitamins.

CONCERNS: Niacin has not been associated with birth defects. Niacin has been assigned a risk factor category of A if used in recommended amounts and a risk factor category of C if used in higher amounts (*see* Appendix 1).

THE BOTTOM LINE: The RDA of niacin is safe in pregnancy.

Nicotine replacement therapy

Nicotine replacement therapy (NRT) is used as an aid in smoking cessation (*see* Smoking; Chewing Tobacco). Nicotine replacement can take the form of a patch that is placed on the skin, pills, inhalers, or chewing gum. These products are sold under the brand names of Commit®, Habitrol®, Nicoderm®, Nicorette®, and Nicotrol®. NRT products can be purchased over-the-counter and no longer require a prescription.

CONCERNS: Nicotine is a powerful drug and one of the most dangerous componenets of tobacco. Researchers have been able to isolate nicotine from breast milk, amniotic fluid, and fetal blood in women who smoked cigarettes or used NRT during pregnancy/lactation. This indicates that the drug can cross the placenta and can enter the breast milk, and therefore the fetus/child is exposed to it as well. Studies have shown an association between nicotine and brain development in experimental animals. Nicotine use during pregnancy has also been associated with learning and behavioral problems, hearing problems, sudden infant death syndrome (SIDS), attention deficit hyperactivity disorder (ADHD), lung problems, and cancer in the offspring. Further, a recent study looking at the psychological benefits of NRT and its usefulness in quitting smoking showed that many people continue to smoke while simultaneously using NRT.

Despite these concerns, the National Health Service of the United Kingdom has extended the use of NRT to pregnant women. Similarly, many health care providers in the United States also prescribe NRT during pregnancy. The justification for this is that pregnant women are exposed to many dangerous chemicals, not just nicotine, while tobacco use is associated with many adverse pregnancy outcomes including ectopic pregnancy, miscarriage, low birth weight, premature rupture of membranes, placenta previa (placenta covering the cervix), placental abruption (premature separation of the placenta from the uterine wall), premature delivery, and preeclampsia (hypertension, protein in the urine, and swelling).

THE BOTTOM LINE: Discuss the risks and benefits of NRT during pregnancy with your health care provider prior to beginning. The safest thing to do is to go "cold turkey."

Nitrates and nitrites

Nitrates are nitrogen-containing compounds that can be found naturally in soil, water, fruits, and vegetables. Nitrates are also used to cure and preserve meats (see Cured meat) such as bacon and hot dogs (see Hot dogs) and are found in cigarette smoke and air pollution. Nitrites are formed from nitrates by bacterial action.

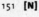

CONCERNS: Women who drank water with high levels of nitrates, secondary to contaminated groundwater, were found to have an increased risk of having an infant with a neural tube defect. Studies in laboratory animals have shown an association between low birth weights and methemoglobinemia (a blood disorder resulting in low oxygen) with diets that are high in nitrates.

Nitrates found in fruits and vegetables do not appear to increase a woman's risk for having a pregnancy complicated by a neural tube defect.

THE BOTTOM LINE: Have your water tested to find out if it is contaminated with dangerous levels of nitrates. Avoid the consumption of nitrate-cured foods, such as hot dogs, bacon, and cured meats.

Nitrofurantoin

Nitrofurantoin is an antibiotic (*see* Antibiotics, oral) that is commonly used in the treatment of urinary tract infections (*see* Urinary tract infections). A brand name for nitrofurantoin is Macrodantin®.

CONCERNS: Nitrofurantoin has been assigned a risk factor category of B (*see* Appendix 1). Nitrofurantoin should not be used after 36 weeks of pregnancy due to a rare but potential complication in the baby (it can cause hemolytic anemia in a fetus with undiagnosed glucose-6-phosphate dehydrogenase deficiency).

THE BOTTOM LINE: Nitrofurantoin is safe prior to 36 weeks of pregnancy.

Nix®

Nix® is a brand name for a head lice shampoo (*see* Head lice).

Nuprin®

Nuprin® is a brand name for ibuprofen (*see* Ibuprofen; Pain relievers).

NutraSweet®

NutraSweet® is a brand name for aspartame (*see* Aspartame; Artificial sweeteners).

Olean® *See* Olestra. ⚠

Olestra ⚠

Olestra, known by the brand name Olean®, is a fat substitute designed to reduce the absorption of calories in fried snacks such as potato chips and tortilla chips. Because the fat in these products is not absorbed by the body, the snacks have fewer calories. Olestra has been introduced due to the increasing concerns over obesity and dieting (*see* Dieting).

CONCERNS: The main concern about Olestra is that since it is not absorbed by the body, vitamins A (*see* Vitamin A), D (*see* Vitamin D), E (*see* Vitamin E), and K (*see* Vitamin K), all fat-soluble vitamins, are also not absorbed. Some nutritionists have expressed concern that during pregnancy, a period when you want adequate intake of vitamins, you may not be getting all the fat-soluble vitamins you need.

Another concern is the possible side effects that some people have experienced from products that contain Olestra, including diarrhea and anal leakage.

THE BOTTOM LINE: Although they are probably safe during pregnancy, products containing Olestra should not be a substitute for eating nutritious foods during pregnancy.

Oils, massage *See* Essential oils.

Omeprazole

Omeprazole, sold under the brand name Prilosec®, is an antacid (*see* Antacids). Omeprazole is classified as a proton pump inhibitor (PPI). PPIs act to block acid secretion from cells in the stomach. Omeprazole is used to treat gastroesophageal reflux disease (GERD).

CONCERNS: Omeprazole has not been associated with any teratogenic (causing birth defects) effects. Omeprazole has been assigned a risk factor category of C (*see* Appendix 1) because it produced dose-related embryonic and fetal mortality in laboratory animals.

THE BOTTOM LINE: Omeprazole appears to be safe in pregnancy at recommended doses.

Oolong tea *See* Tea.

Oxycodone

Oxycodone, sold under the brand name OxyContin®, is a narcotic pain reliever (*see* Pain relievers).

CONCERNS: Oxycodone has been assigned a risk factor category of B when used in prescribed doses and a risk factor category of D (*see* Appendix 1) when used for long periods or close to delivery. No association with birth defects has been seen with the use of this drug.

THE BOTTOM LINE: Oxycodone is safe to take as prescribed during pregnancy. Avoid use for long periods or close to delivery.

OxyContin®

OxyContin® is a brand name for oxycodone (*see* Oxycodone).

Pain relievers   ⚠ ∴

Most pain relievers are characterized as nonsteroidal anti-inflammatory drugs (NSAIDs) (*see* Aspirin; Ibuprofen; Naproxen), acetaminophen (*see* Acetaminophen), or narcotics (*see* Codeine; Oxycodone).

CONCERNS:

- *NSAIDs:* Although ibuprofen and naproxen have been assigned a risk factor category of B in the first two trimesters, it is recommended that you avoid these drugs throughout pregnancy, but especially in the third trimester. A recent review of over 36,000 women who took NSAIDs in the first trimester showed an association between NSAID use and birth defects. This study showed that 7 percent of these women had a baby with at least one malformation. If future research confirms these findings, the U.S. Food and Drug Administration (FDA) may need to change the risk factor category of these medications.

- *Acetaminophen:* Acetaminophen is considered to be the safest pain reliever in pregnancy. It is viewed as the pain reliever of choice in pregnancy.

- *Narcotics:* Most narcotic pain relievers are considered to be safe in pregnancy when used as prescribed. However, there is a risk of neonatal withdrawal if used for prolonged periods or close to delivery. These drugs should be used cautiously and only as directed.

THE BOTTOM LINE: Most pain relievers are safe during pregnancy. Take only as directed and make sure that your health care provider knows that you are pregnant. If you have any concerns about abuse of these medications, please discuss them with your doctor.

Paint fumes ⚠

Paint fumes are odorous gases that come from the liquid solvent, or vehicle, that is used to suspend the pigments in paint.

CONCERNS: Many of the solvents used in paint are known to be dangerous. However, it is difficult to quantify how much of the chemical gases are actually inhaled into your system. As such, studies have shown mixed results.

Exposure to organic solvents has been associated with an increased rate of miscarriage, cancer, and immune problems (*see* Benzene). A recent study found that children of women exposed to common organic solvents during pregnancy also had significantly lower scores on a wide range of cognitive, motor, and behavioral tests.

Studies from women who sniffed paint, as a form of drug abuse, during their pregnancy showed an increased incidence of children born with features similar to those seen in fetal alcohol syndrome infants. Women who had an occupational exposure to paint did not appear to have a higher rate of miscarriage. One could extrapolate that women with an occasional exposure to painting would have a lower risk than those who sniffed paint or used it occupationally.

THE BOTTOM LINE: Data are limited regarding the effects of paint fumes during pregnancy. By wearing protective clothing and using a mask, you can significantly decrease your exposure. Try to paint in a well-ventilated area and don't work near foods. Try to avoid spray paints, as their use will release more paint particles into the air than brush-on paint. Use latex paint when possible, as opposed to oil-based paints, as they have the lowest concentration of organic solvents. Avoiding painting altogether will eliminate the risks.

Pamelor® ⊘

Pamelor® is a brand name for nortriptyline (*see* Psychiatric medications).

Panalol®

Panalol® is a brand name for acetaminophen (*see* Acetaminophen; Pain relievers).

Parasites

Parasites are organisms that live inside the body and may cause disease. Examples include *Toxoplasmosis* (*see* Toxoplasmosis), *Trichomonas* (*see* Trichomoniasis), and intestinal parasites.

CONCERNS: Some common parasites, such as *Toxoplasmosis*, are more dangerous than others during pregnancy. *Toxoplasmosis* infection can cause fetal death, preterm labor, and some kinds of birth defects. However, *Toxoplasmosis* is a common childhood infection. Many people are immune to it, and a quick blood test from your health care provider will reveal whether you are immune. If you are immune, there is no need to worry. If you are susceptible to *Toxoplasmosis*, use caution when changing cat litter (*see* Litter boxes), while gardening (*see* Gardening), and while eating and preparing raw or undercooked meat (*see* Cured meat; Deli meats, cooked and uncooked).

Trichomonas is another parasite that can be dangerous during pregnancy. *Trichomonas* can cause a vaginal infection that can be asymptomatic or may be associated with vaginal discharge and odor. It should be treated during pregnancy because it has been associated with an increased risk of preterm labor and premature rupture of membranes.

Intestinal parasites can be acquired through eating contaminated food or drinking water. Symptoms include diarrhea, nausea and vomiting, stomach pain, weight loss, and fatigue. Intestinal parasites can be more dangerous during pregnancy because the infection can prevent you from absorbing all the nutrients that your baby needs, and this will put you at risk for having a low-birth-weight baby.

THE BOTTOM LINE: The term *parasitic infections* encompasses a variety of infections, some of which are dangerous during pregnancy. Please consult your health care provider regarding specific infections and their treatments.

⚠️

Pâté

Pâté is made from seasoned ground meat and can be smooth or chunky. It may be served hot or cold and is generally served as an appetizer. There are several variations including one made of foie gras (*see* Foie gras), one made in a mold lined with pork fat called a terrine, and one cooked in a bread crust called pâté en croûte. Pâtés are generally made from pork, veal, liver, fish, or poultry; vegetables; and seasonings.

CONCERNS: A study in 2001 by the Food Safety and Inspection Service of the United States Department of Agriculture (FSIS/USDA) determined that many pregnant women were either not aware of the dangers of certain foods or did not handle these foods properly in the home. It is important to know that you are at risk for several food-borne illnesses that can be contracted through prepared meats (*see* Deli meats, cooked and uncooked) during pregnancy.

Pâtés are susceptible to *Listeria* (*see* Listeria) from contamination by meat slicers, cutting boards (*see* Cutting boards), knives, and refrigerators. Even if pâtés are properly refrigerated, this bacterium may still be present. Although you won't completely eliminate the risks, the USDA recommends that precooked meats should be properly stored below 40°F/4.5°C and should be thrown away if they have an expired freshness date.

THE BOTTOM LINE: The USDA and the U.S. Food and Drug Administration (FDA) recommend that pregnant women don't eat refrigerated pâté and meat spreads. Only canned pâté that has been opened that day and meat spreads that do not require refrigeration are safe.

Paxil®

⚠️

Paxil® is a brand name for paroxetine (*see* Psychiatric medications).

Peanuts

⚠️

Peanuts are a legume high in protein and fat. They are the main component of peanut butter and peanut oil. They may be purchased raw, roasted, or boiled, and may be salted or unsalted.

CONCERNS: Peanut allergy affects approximately 1 out of every 200 four-year-olds. In order to develop an allergy, a person must be exposed to that allergen. Some researchers have begun to consider that this exposure may first occur in utero or during breastfeeding. Some health care providers have begun to recommend that women avoid eating peanuts during pregnancy and breastfeeding, especially if there is a history of allergies in the family. Some studies have shown that the chance that a child will have an allergy to peanuts increases with the amount of peanuts consumed during pregnancy.

A toxin called aflatoxin can be produced by a fungus that grows on peanuts. There are not enough data on this toxin to advise avoiding peanuts during pregnancy, due to worry over aflatoxin.

THE BOTTOM LINE: There are not enough data to suggest that all pregnant and nursing women should avoid eating all peanut products. However, there may be an association between eating peanuts and peanut allergy in children. Consider avoiding peanuts if you have a significant history of allergies in your family.

Pedicures See Manicures.

Penicillin
Penicillin is an antibiotic (*see* Antibiotics, oral).
CONCERNS: Penicillin has been assigned a risk factor category of B (*see* Appendix 1).
THE BOTTOM LINE: Penicillin is safe for use during pregnancy.

Pepto Bismol®
Pepto Bismol® is a brand name of bismuth subsalicylate compound (*see* Bismuth subsalicylate).

Perms
A "perm," or permanent, is a process of using chemicals to permanently curl hair.
CONCERNS: Many chemicals can be absorbed through the skin and pass from the mother to the baby's bloodstream. It is well known that certain chemicals can cause birth defects.

THE BOTTOM LINE: There is limited information on permanents during pregnancy. However, it is unlikely that significant amounts of chemicals are absorbed into the skin. No information associating perms with pregnancy complications was found. If you decide to get a perm, wait until after the first trimester, when the baby's organs have formed.

Pesticides ⊘

Pesticides are chemicals used to kill insects, such as fleas, mosquitoes, ants, cockroaches, and animals, including rodents. Pesticides can be obtained in the form of sprays (*see* Insect repellents; Insecticides), creams, or animal collars (*see* Flea and tick medication). The active chemical in the most effective insect repellents is diethyltoluamide, better known as DEET (*see* DEET).

CONCERNS: The use of insect repellents has increased because of concern over mosquitoes that transmit West Nile disease and ticks that transmit Lyme disease. Concern over the use of DEET increased after several reports of seizures in young children exposed to DEET. DEET is also known to be absorbed through the skin and can cross the placenta in animal studies. There is limited information about DEET use during pregnancy. However, in one known case, a child born to a woman who used DEET throughout her pregnancy had birth defects. Overall, DEET is considered to be safe for use during pregnancy. Please see the DEET entry for complete safety recommendations.

Women living one-quarter mile from agricultural crops sprayed with insecticides appear 1.5 times more likely to have a baby with a birth defect. Insecticides have also been associated with attention deficit hyperactivity disorder (ADHD).

THE BOTTOM LINE: The safest thing to do is to avoid all pesticides throughout your pregnancy and especially during the first trimester. There appears to be an increased risk of birth defects with early and prolonged exposure. If you must use these products, limit your exposure by having someone else do the spraying, staying out of the room for the directed amount of time, wearing gloves and a mask, and using in well-ventilated areas. If your skin is inadvertently exposed to insecticides or if they are ingested, call poison control.

Pet rodents ⊘

Pet rodents include mice, hamsters, and guinea pigs. Laboratory animals could also be included in this category.

CONCERNS: Wild mice have been found to carry lymphocytic chori-omeningitis virus (LCMV). They can contaminate domesticated mice (including laboratory mice and pet mice), hamsters, and guinea pigs in breeding facilities. This virus can be transmitted to humans through contact with infected urine, body fluids, droppings, and nesting material, and through inhalation of droplets or dust containing the virus. The virus has been shown to be able to cross the placenta and can cause fetal death and severe birth defects such as mental retardation, brain abnormalities, and vision problems. Approximately 5 percent of the total population has antibodies for this virus, indicating a prior infection or exposure.

THE BOTTOM LINE: Currently there is no treatment available for LCMV, so you should avoid contact with pet rodents prior to and during pregnancy and avoid cleaning any droppings from wild rodents. If you do come in contact with wild rodent droppings, wash your hands carefully.

Phazyme® ✓

Phazyme® is a brand of simethicone (*see* Simethicone).

Phosphorus ⚠

Phosphorus is an essential mineral that is a major component of bones. It is generally found in the form of a phosphate. It can be found in dairy products, poultry, eggs, grains, and legumes.

CONCERNS: A high intake of phosphorus has been associated with a decreased ability to absorb calcium. Since supplemental phosphorus is categorized as a food supplement, it is not regulated by the U.S. Food and Drug Administration. Thus, there is no guarantee of the strength, purity, or safety of this product. You should inform your health care provider if you are taking any nutritional supplements.

Phosphorus deficiency is rare, since phosphorus is plentiful in many foods. Deficiency can occur in diabetes, malnutrition, alcohol abuse, and high-dose antacid use. Since phosphorus is a major component of bones, untreated phosphorus deficiency could lead to bone fractures.

THE BOTTOM LINE: Phosphorus deficiency is rare and supplementation is probably not necessary during pregnancy.

Phthalates

Phthalates are compounds used in plastics and personal care products. They make plastics more pliable. They are commonly used in bags, medical equipment, toys, paints and building supplies (*see* Building materials), cosmetics, soaps and shampoos, and pesticides (*see* Pesticides).

CONCERNS: Phthalates can accumulate in the body fat of humans and animals. Their structure is similar to estrogen, and therefore researchers have speculated that exposure during pregnancy may affect the developing fetus. A recent study showed that exposure to phthalates during human pregnancy was associated with smaller penis size and incomplete testicular descent in boys. Similar problems including decreased sperm counts have also been seen in studies using laboratory animals. Occupational exposure has been associated with miscarriage. Phthalates have also been implicated in the development of childhood asthma and allergies. Phthalates have been isolated from baby formula, drinking water, house dust, and dairy products. However, there is little agreement as to whether average exposure will lead to health problems.

In 1998 the U.S. Consumer Product Safety Commission (CPSC) looked at the association between phthalates (diisononyl phthalate or DINP) used in children's teethers and rattles and resultant health problems. They concluded that the risks were low but requested that manufacturers of these items should discontinue using DINP in these products by 1999. Arco Toys, Chicco, Disney, Evenflo, The First Years, Gerber, Hasbro (Playskool), Little Tykes, Mattel (Fisher-Price), Safety 1st, Sassy, Shelcore Toys, and Tyco Preschool have all complied with this request.

Dibutyl phthalate (DBP), dimethyl phthalate (DMP), and diethyl phthalate (DEP) are phthlates used in nail polish (*see* Nail polish), hair sprays, perfumes, and other cosmetics. The FDA requires that under the Fair Packaging and Labeling Act (FPLA) cosmetics must list their ingredients. However, it is often impossible to get this information as some ingredients, such as fragrance, do not require a complete listing of all the individual ingredients (i.e., the label will just list "fragrance"). The FDA is continuing to monitor cosmetics, and this issue became a program priority item in 2004.

THE BOTTOM LINE: Until more is known, avoid excessive exposure to phthalates during pregnancy. Read product labels carefully and try to avoid cosmetics that contain DBP, DMP, and DEP. Purchase toys that say "phthalate free" or use latex or silicone instead. Discard any soft plastic toys made before 1999, especially if the materials are unknown. Watch for any changing recommendations made by the FDA.

Piercings

Piercing involves puncturing the skin and placing an object, usually metal, to maintain the opening and provide decoration. Piercings can be done on any part of the body, but most commonly they are done in the earlobes, face, and belly, and less commonly in the nipples of the breasts and in the genitals.

CONCERNS: The main concern over piercing during pregnancy centers on the risk of infection. If you already have a piercing it is probably fine to leave it as it is unless it is causing discomfort. If you have a belly ring, your expanding abdomen could cause it to stretch and the ring may become uncomfortable. You can remove the ring if this occurs; otherwise it should be treated as you normally would. Genital jewelry can be removed or left in depending on your desires and personal preferences and any concern with trauma at the time of delivery. Nipple rings should be removed if nursing because of the theoretical risk of aspiration during breast feeding.

THE BOTTOM LINE: Although there are no scientific studies examining these issues, common sense tells us to avoid practices that could cause an infection during pregnancy. If you already have a piercing, no special precautions need to be taken unless you are experiencing any discomfort.

Pilates

Pilates is a form of exercise (see Exercise) that involves strengthening the core muscles (abdomen, back, and pelvis) through a series of postures and stretches. Providers of Pilates during pregnancy state that the benefits include increased energy levels, increased speed of recovery following delivery, decreased pain and tension in muscles as postural changes occur, and increased circulation.

CONCERNS: Although no scientific studies looking specifically at the effects of Pilates during pregnancy could be found, exercise is encouraged during pregnancy. Regular exercise has been associated with prevention of gestational diabetes (diabetes related to pregnancy), controlling weight gain, and maternal well-being. It seems like good common sense to follow the same guidelines that yoga (see Yoga) instructors offer to their pregnant clients. This advice includes avoiding prolonged poses on the back, as the weight of the fetus pressing against the aorta (a major artery) can restrict the blood flow to the lower body, including the uterus. If you feel dizzy or light-headed while on your back, immediately bend your knees and slowly roll over to your side. Avoid poses that stretch the muscles too much, particularly the abdominal muscles. You are more apt to tear and strain muscles now because the amount of the hormone relaxin in the blood increases. Relaxin is a hormone produced by the reproductive tract during pregnancy. Its main role is to inhibit uterine contractions, soften the cervix, and dilate blood vessels. Relaxin also works on other tissues such as ligaments and can make it easier to strain muscles and ligaments while exercising. Avoid all postures that put pressure on your abdomen, especially forward folds, twists, and belly-down postures. Listen carefully to your body. If you feel any discomfort, stop. You will probably need to adapt most postures to your body's physical changes. You may wish to restrict yourself to classes specifically labeled prenatal.

THE BOTTOM LINE: With certain precautions, Pilates appears to be safe during pregnancy.

Polyvinyl chloride plastic (PVC)

Polyvinyl chloride plastic (PVC) is a common plastic used to make vinyl, luggage, shower curtains, toys, pipes, and bottles.

CONCERNS: PVC plastic releases dioxin when produced or burned. Dioxin has been shown to be a carcinogenic and can also harm the immune and reproductive systems. PVC can also release variable amounts of mercury (*see* Mercury) and phthalates (*see* Phthalates), which are known to be toxic to humans. A 2005 study demonstrated a link between exposure to PVC during pregnancy and adverse effects in male offspring.

In 2005 the Center for Health, Environment and Justice (CHEJ) worked with several companies to encourage them to discontinue using PVC in their products and packaging.

THE BOTTOM LINE: It is unclear how much exposure to PVC is safe during pregnancy, but a recent study has demonstrated a link to adverse effects. Try to avoid purchasing products made with PVC as identified by the "V" and/or "3" in the recycle symbol. These products cannot be recycled and are a threat to the environment.

Pools

Swimming pool water is generally treated with a variety of chemicals, including chlorine (*see* Chlorine), to destroy harmful bacteria.

CONCERNS: A few studies have found that a group of by-products of chlorine, trihalomethanes (THMs), can be found in water treated with chlorine and is associated with low birth weight and fetal birth defects such as neural tube defects. THMs can be absorbed through the skin and lungs. It is unclear what levels are dangerous during pregnancy. Other studies have not found this association. Chlorine can also break down to chloroform, which may also cause harm during a pregnancy. The Environmental Protection Agency (EPA) has set up standards to monitor these levels and is continuing to do research on this issue.

THE BOTTOM LINE: Until more is known about the chemicals used in pool water, we must depend on the EPA to ensure our safety. If newer research confirms the reports of increased birth defects from swimming in water with high THMs, stricter standards and testing will need to be implemented. THM levels have been shown to be higher in pool water during busy use, so try to swim when the pool is less crowded. Outdoor pools and pools with high ceilings may have lower levels of THMs in the air and may be a safer option. Rinse off any chemicals after you leave the pool.

Poppy seeds ☑

Poppy seeds are the small grayish seeds from the poppy plant. They are dried and added to foods for a crunchy texture and a nutty flavor. They are rich in protein and fat.

CONCERNS: Because poppy seeds come from the poppy plant, the source of morphine and opium, there is some concern over the amount of active compounds that might be ingested by eating these seeds.

THE BOTTOM LINE: The poppy seed is generally regarded as safe when used for food.

Potassium ☑

Potassium is a mineral or electrolyte that is found in all cells of the body. Electrolytes are important for the proper functioning of the cells, for transport of material to and from the cells, and for nerve conduction, water balance, and muscle contraction. The kidneys are responsible for keeping potassium levels stable, and excess potassium is secreted into the urine. Low levels of potassium are associated with diarrhea, vomiting, and certain medications, such as diuretics. Potassium is found in many foods, including dark leafy green vegetables, tomatoes, potatoes, oranges, bananas, whole grains, and fish.

CONCERNS: Potassium levels are one of the things that are checked when your doctor orders a complete blood chemistry (CBC) profile. However, potassium levels are not routinely checked unless you have a condition that puts you at increased risk for having abnormal potassium levels.

THE BOTTOM LINE: Potassium deficiency is rare. Excess potassium will be secreted into your urine through the kidneys unless you have kidney disease. There is no need to supplement your diet during pregnancy unless you are taking certain medications or it is recommended by your health care provider.

Prenatal vitamins *See* Multivitamins.

Preparation H®

Preparation H® is a brand name for a hemorrhoid medication (*see* Hemorrhoid medications).

Prescription medications

Prescription medications are drugs that require a prescription from a physician prior to their use. They include antibiotics (*see* Antibiotics), antifungal medications (*see* Antifungal medications, oral and topical), and certain pain medications (*see* Pain relievers).

CONCERNS: Make sure your health care provider knows that you are pregnant and prescribes a drug with a risk factor category of A, B, or C (*see* Appendix 1).

THE BOTTOM LINE: Consult with your health care provider prior to taking prescription drugs during pregnancy. Many are safe, but some are dangerous and can cause birth defects. If you take any long-term medications, inform your OB/GYN ASAP.

Prevacid®

Prevacid® is a brand name for lansoprazole (*see* Antacids; Lansoprazole).

Prilosec®

Prilosec® is a brand name for omeprazole (*see* Omeprazole; Antacids).

Probiotics

Probiotics are live bacteria and yeast, most commonly the bacteria *Lactobacillus* and the yeast *Saccharomyces*, which are consumed orally and then live with preexisting bacteria. Probiotics need to be replenished constantly. An example of a probiotic is *Lactobacillus acidophilus* (*see* Acidophilus; Yogurt). Lactobacillus can be consumed in pill or capsule form, in yogurt with live cultures, or as a vaginal suppository to treat yeast infections.

CONCERNS: A study from Finland found that giving probiotics during pregnancy and breastfeeding helped to reduce the incidence of atopic eczema during the first two years of life. In this study, the probiotic used was identified as *Lactobacillus rhamnosus*. The study failed to find any significant differences in the incidence of allergic rhinitis or asthma.

Since probiotics are categorized as a food supplements, they are not regulated by the Food and Drug Administration. Thus, there is no guarantee of the strength, purity, or safety of these products. You should inform your health care provider if you are taking any nutritional supplements. If you are at risk for preterm labor, you should avoid using vaginal suppositories unless directed by your physician.

THE BOTTOM LINE: No adverse effects following probiotic use has been found during pregnancy. More research will need to be done before we can document the safety and usefulness of probiotics.

Progesterone

Progesterone is a hormone that is necessary for pregnancy. During the first 10 weeks of pregnancy, most of the progesterone is made by the corpus luteum in the ovary. After that, the placenta is the main producer of progesterone. Synthetic progesterone is used in hormonal birth control and in hormone replacement therapy.

Recent evidence has shown that progesterone may help prevent pregnancy loss and preterm labor. One recent study showed an association between progesterone supplementation in high-risk pregnancies and a decreased incidence in preterm births. According to some evidence, women with low progesterone levels during early pregnancy may benefit from added progesterone. In this condition, called a corpus luteal defect, the corpus luteum on the ovary that normally secretes progesterone during the first 10 weeks is not functioning well. However, data are controversial. Progesterone supplementation has been used during early pregnancy in women who have no ovarian function as a result of having their ovaries removed due to an ovarian cyst or mass.

CONCERNS: Since birth control pills have been assigned a risk factor category X (*see* Appendix 1), many women are concerned about taking progesterone during pregnancy. However, studies have failed to show any clear teratogenic (cause of birth defects) effects due to progesterone use during pregnancy.

THE BOTTOM LINE: Progesterone appears to be safe during pregnancy. However, it should be taken only if recommended by your health care provider.

Prolonged standing ⚠

Prolonged standing is defined as standing for more than three hours in a day.

CONCERNS: A study from Thailand found an association between standing longer than three hours per day and an increased incidence of preterm birth.

The American Medical Association recommends that women do not spend more than four continuous hours a day on their feet after the twenty-fourth week of pregnancy and not more than 30 minutes after the thirty-second week. Discuss the need to make these changes with your employer. Employers should make every effort to accommodate your needs when possible, or you may need to consider going on disability leave.

THE BOTTOM LINE: Prolonged standing during pregnancy has been associated with preterm labor and preterm contractions. If your job requires this, you may need to consider going on disability or changing your work habits temporarily.

Prophylactic antibiotics ⚠

Occasionally, you may have a condition during pregnancy that requires prophylactic, or preventive, antibiotics (see Antibiotics, oral). Examples of this may be certain heart conditions or being a carrier of group B strep (GBS).

CONCERNS: Each antibiotic/antimicrobial has an individual risk factor category. Most are perfectly safe in pregnancy, but some should be avoided. Make sure your health care provider knows that you are pregnant and prescribes a drug with a risk factor category of A, B, or C (see Appendix 1).

THE BOTTOM LINE: Prophylactic antibiotics may be recommended by your health care provider for a variety or reasons. Most antibiotics are safe during pregnancy.

Prozac®

Prozac® is a brand name for fluoxetine (*see* Psychiatric medications).

Pseudoephedrine

Pseudoephedrine is a popular decongestant (*see* Decongestants) found in many cold remedies (*see* Cough and cold medicines).

CONCERNS: Because pseudoephedrine is often used in combination with other medicines, it has been difficult to sort out its effects on pregnancy. Pseudoephedrine has been assigned a risk factor category of C (*see* Appendix 1).

THE BOTTOM LINE: When used as directed, pseudoephedrine appears to be safe during pregnancy.

Psychiatric medications

Psychiatric disorders are common in women of reproductive age. These disorders include depression, bipolar disorder, psychosis, anxiety, and substance abuse. Medications include antidepressants, antipsychotics, sedatives, anxiolytics, drugs of abuse, and mood stabilizers.

CONCERNS: It was previously thought that psychiatric medications should be avoided during pregnancy to prevent possible birth defects, but information about their risks and benefits proves that many can be taken safely throughout pregnancy. A recent study showed an association between maternal depression at any time between 1 year prior and 9 years after giving birth and attention deficit hyperactivity disorder (ADHD). Therefore it may be wise to treat depression during pregnancy.

- *Antidepressants:* Antidepressants are generally categorized as tricyclic antidepressants (TCAs) or as selective serotonin reuptake inhibitors (SSRIs). TCAs include Elavil® (amitriptyline) and Pamelor® (nortriptyline), which have both been assigned a risk factor category of D (*see* Appendix 1). These drugs have not been associated with any major birth defects but do put the newborn at risk for irritability, seizures, jitteriness, and tachycardia (fast heart rate). SSRIs include Paxil® (paroxetine), Prozac® (fluoxetine), Wellbutrin®. (bupropion), and Zoloft® (sertraline). SSRIs are not generally associated with any birth defects but can cause agitation and tachycardia (rapid heartbeat) in newborns. These SSRIs all have been assigned a risk factor category of B. One recent study noted convulsions and withdrawal syndrome in newborns of women who used SSRIs. Recently, a risk of major congenital birth defects in infants born to women taking Paxil has been identified. Newer studies have shown that both sertraline and paroxetine have been associated with birth defects. However, the absolute risks are thought to be small.

- *Antipsychotics:* Antipsychotics are generally assigned risk factor categories of B and C. Examples include Haldol® (haloperidol). These drugs are further categorized as low-potency agents and high-potency agents. High-potency agents, such as haloperidol, have not been associated with any congenital malformations and are considered the drugs of choice in pregnancy.
- *Sedatives:* Ambien® (zolpidem) has been assigned a risk factor category of B. There are no reports of adverse fetal effects in mothers who used zolpidem.
- *Anxiolytics:* Anxiolytics, or antianxiety medications, have been assigned risk factor categories of C, D, and X. It is generally recommended that you stop using these drugs prior to conception, as they have been associated with orofacial cleft and hypotonia (decreased muscle tone), hypothermia (decreased body temperature), and apnea (breathing problems) in the newborn. If you need to use these drugs, avoid taking them in the first trimester and around the time of birth. Common anxiolytics include Ativan® (lorazepam), Librium® (chlordiazepoxide), Valium® (diazepam), and Xanax® (alprazolam). Xanax and Valium® have a risk factor category of X.

- *Drugs of abuse: See* Drugs of abuse.
- *Mood stabilizers:* Lithium has a risk factor category of D and has been associated with fetal heart abnormalities as well as hypotonia in the newborn.

THE BOTTOM LINE: Many psychiatric medicines are safe during pregnancy and should be taken to maintain the health of the mother, but some should be avoided. Consider consulting with your OB/GYN and therapist prior to pregnancy to see if you need to switch to a safer medication.

PVC *See* Polyvinyl chloride plastic.

Pyridoxine

Pyridoxine, or Vitamin B_6, is a water-soluble B complex vitamin. The recommended daily allowance (RDA) during pregnancy is 2.2 milligrams. Pyridoxine can be found in fish, poultry, liver, avocados, bananas, carrots, corn, nuts, legumes, whole-grain cereals, and multivitamins (*see* Multivitamins).

CONCERNS: Vitamin B_6 has been shown to decrease nausea related to pregnancy. Deficiency of Vitamin B_6 has been associated with several pregnancy complications, including nausea and vomiting, preeclampsia (hypertension, protein in the urine, and swelling), and fetal convulsions. High doses have not been associated with birth defects. Pyridoxine has been assigned a risk factor category of A (*see* Appendix 1).

THE BOTTOM LINE: The RDA of pyridoxine is safe during pregnancy. Several studies report that it helps decrease nausea and vomiting related to pregnancy.

Raw fish *See* Sushi. ⚠

Red Bull® ⚠

Red Bull® is a brand name for an energy drink (*see* Energy drinks).

Red tea *See* Tea. ⚠

Reptiles ⚠

Reptiles are cold-blooded, egg-laying, vertebrate animals. They include lizards, snakes, crocodiles, and turtles.

CONCERNS: As many as 90 percent of reptiles can carry a bacterium called *Salmonella* (*see Salmonella*). *Salmonella* can cause diarrhea, fever, and abdominal pain. It is most dangerous in people who have a weakened immune system. Women who are pregnant do not appear to be at an increased risk of getting *Salmonella*. However, one type of this bacterium can cross the placenta and cause miscarriage, stillbirth, and preterm labor. According to the Centers for Disease Control and Prevention (CDC), reptiles are responsible for 70,000 to 90,000 cases of *Salmonella* infections per year.

If you have reptiles as pets, the CDC recommends these precautions:

- Wash hands after handling the reptile or the cage.
- Do not allow reptiles in areas where food is prepared or consumed.

- Do not wash cages in the kitchen sink.
- Carefully disinfect areas used to clean the cage with bleach.
- Do not let animals roam freely about the home.
- If you are expecting a child, remove the reptile from the house before the infant arrives.
- Keep reptiles away from children younger than five years of age and away from people with weakened immune systems.
- Day care centers should not house reptiles.

THE BOTTOM LINE: Reptiles carry *Salmonella*, which can be dangerous during pregnancy, early childhood, and in cases of a weakened immune system. Therefore, it seems reasonable to remove these pets from the home while pregnant. Precautions will help to reduce the risk of acquiring a *Salmonella* infection during pregnancy.

Retin-A®

Retin-A is the brand name for tretinoin (*see* Tretinoin).

Riboflavin

Riboflavin, or Vitamin B₂, is a water-soluble B complex vitamin. The recommended daily allowance (RDA) of riboflavin during pregnancy is 1.6 milligrams. Riboflavin can be found in meat, poultry, organ meats, eggs, dairy products, leafy green vegetables, wheat germ, and multivitamins (*see* Multivitamins). Riboflavin deficiency is rare in the United States.

CONCERNS: Riboflavin has been assigned a risk factor category of A if used in recommended amounts and a risk factor category of C if used in amounts above the RDA (*see* Appendix 1).

THE BOTTOM LINE: The RDA of riboflavin is safe during pregnancy.

Rolaids®

Rolaids® is a brand name for an antacid (*see* Antacids).

Running

The American College of Obstetrics and Gynecology recommends 30 minutes of exercise on most days during pregnancy (*see* Exercise).

CONCERNS: Several studies on running during pregnancy failed to show any adverse pregnancy outcomes. Common sense is important here, and there are a few things you need to be aware of. First, it seems to be very important that you take the time to stretch. During pregnancy, the amount of the hormone relaxin in the blood increases. Relaxin is a hormone produced by the reproductive tract during pregnancy. Its main role is to inhibit uterine contractions, soften the cervix, and dilate blood vessels. Relaxin also works on other tissues such as ligaments and can make it easier to strain muscles and ligaments while exercising. Listen to your body. If you are having pain, you may want to slow down. You may need to urinate more frequently, requiring some planning when on a longer run. A new sports bra may be in order due to the changing size and sensitivity of your breasts. As your body changes as your baby grows, you may find that you need to slow down or shorten your runs. Be careful to keep well hydrated and avoid becoming overheated, as this has been associated with preterm contractions.

It is generally felt that it is safe to continue with your regular running routine throughout pregnancy. However, starting a new exercise regimen while pregnant is not recommended. Many women can continue to run throughout their entire pregnancy, while some find it uncomfortable and need to slow down as their due date approaches.

THE BOTTOM LINE: Studies have not shown any adverse effects from running during pregnancy. Use common sense and slow down if you are experiencing pain, contractions, dizziness, or vaginal bleeding, and don't forget to stretch. If you have any concerns, please discuss these with your OB/GYN.

Saccharin ⚠️

Saccharin is an artificial sweetener (*see* Artificial sweeteners). It is found in many diet drinks and diet foods.

CONCERNS: Saccharin has been assigned a risk factor category of C (*see* Appendix 1). The Food and Drug Administration considers saccharin a food additive that may be dangerous in humans and should be avoided during pregnancy. Saccharin is thought to be a low-level carcinogen (cancer causing) and should be avoided, even when not pregnant.

THE BOTTOM LINE: Until more is known about the effects of saccharin during pregnancy, limit your intake of this product.

Salads ⚠️

Salads are generally made from raw greens, lettuce, herbs, and other raw vegetables or fruit and topped with a dressing. The term *salads* can also refer to dishes that are made from chopped meat, eggs, or seafood, fruit, or pasta mixed with a vinaigrette or mayonnaise (*see* Homemade mayonnaise), such as tuna, chicken, egg (*see* Eggs), or pasta salad.

CONCERNS: Raw foods can become contaminated with many bacteria, including *Escherichia coli* (*see* E. coli infection), *Campylobacter* (*see* Campylobacter), or *Salmonella* (*see* Salmonella). Contamination can occur when vegetables are grown in areas with improperly treated water or through human contamination. To avoid becoming ill from salads made with raw vegetables, wash fruits and vegetables carefully in water and avoid foods that can be contaminated with *E. coli*, such as raw sprouts (*see* Sprouts, raw). Avoid raw salads from establishments that do not have good sanitation. Salads made with homemade mayonnaise (*see* Homemade mayonnaise) can be contaminated with *Salmonella*.

THE BOTTOM LINE: Raw foods can be contaminated with different types of bacteria. The safest thing is to wash vegetables carefully or eat them cooked. Avoid homemade mayonnaise unless it is prepared with pasteurized eggs.

Salmonella

Salmonella is a bacterium that can cause diarrhea, fever, and abdominal pain. It is most dangerous in people who have a weakened immune system. *Salmonella* is known to contaminate eggs (*see* Eggs), poultry, alfalfa sprouts (*see* Sprouts, raw), and reptiles (*see* Reptiles).

CONCERNS: Women who are pregnant do not appear to be at an increased risk of getting *Salmonella*. However, one type of this bacterium can cross the placenta and cause miscarriage, stillbirth, and preterm labor. *Salmonella* does not appear to cause birth defects.

THE BOTTOM LINE: If you are concerned about *Salmonella* during your pregnancy, it is probably best to avoid raw eggs, foods containing raw eggs (*see* Cookie dough; Eggnog; Homemade ice cream; Homemade mayonnaise), and undercooked poultry. Wash your hands frequently when cooking with raw eggs or poultry and clean knives and cutting boards (*see* Cutting boards) properly to avoid cross-contamination. Cooking any food to 165°F/74°C will destroy Salmonella. Using pasteurized eggs in homemade mayonnaise and eggnog will eliminate the concern over raw eggs. Store eggs properly below 40°F/4.5°C and use before their freshness date passes.

SAM-e

SAM-e, or S-Adenosylmethionine, is a chemical made naturally in the body from the amino acid methionine. A deficiency in this amino acid is thought to cause a deficiency in SAM-e, which has been associated with depression, osteoarthritis, and liver disorders. Consequently, SAM-e is used to treat depression, fibromyalgia, liver disease, and migraine headaches. SAM-e can be purchased as a food supplement in pill form.

CONCERNS: Since SAM-e is classified as a food supplement, it is not regulated by the U.S. Food and Drug Administration (FDA). Thus, there is no guarantee as to the strength, purity, or effectiveness of this product. You should inform your health care provider if you are taking any supplements.

THE BOTTOM LINE: Since SAM-e supplements are not approved by the FDA, they are not recommended for use during pregnancy. However, these supplements have been used in Europe for many years and have not been associated with adverse pregnancy outcomes.

Saunas ⚠️

Saunas are rooms that are heated with dry heat for the purpose of relaxation. They are often found in health clubs (*see* Health clubs).

CONCERNS: Concern over the use of saunas has centered on worry over increasing maternal core body temperature (CBT). Numerous studies have made an association between elevated temperatures and the increased incidence of neural tube defects and miscarriages. Saunas appear to be dangerous if your core body temperature (CBT) rises to 102.5°F/39°C. Some researchers have suggested that if a pregnant woman's CBT becomes that high, she would feel uncomfortable and get out of the sauna.

Time spent in a sauna could also result in dehydration, which can make you feel light-headed.

THE BOTTOM LINE: Saunas are not recommended during pregnancy.

Scuba diving ⚠️

Scuba diving is diving under water with supplemental oxygen.

CONCERNS: The main concerns about scuba diving during pregnancy is related to the risks of decompression sickness.

THE BOTTOM LINE: Scuba diving is not recommended during pregnancy despite limited data associating it with adverse pregnancy outcomes.

Seafood

Seafood refers to any edible fish or animal that comes from the sea (*see* Fish; Shellfish; Smoked fish; Sushi).

Seat belts

Seat belts are now standard in new cars and have been proven to reduce death and injury during car accidents.

CONCERNS: A recent study showed that many pregnant women do not wear seat belts due to concerns about damage to the baby, should they get into an accident. In fact, pregnant women who are not wearing seat belts and suffer a car accident are three times more likely to experience a fatal injury to the fetus and two times more likely to have excessive maternal bleeding.

THE BOTTOM LINE: The American College of Obstetrics and Gynecology recommends that all pregnant women wear seat belts while driving. Ideally the seat belt should be a lap and shoulder combination. The lap portion should fit snugly under the woman's abdomen and the shoulder strap diagonally across her chest.

Secondhand smoke

Secondhand smoke is the smoke you are exposed to when other people are smoking cigarettes, cigars, or pipes.

CONCERNS: Attention to the dangers of secondhand smoke has been evident from recent legislation prohibiting smoking in public areas.

Babies who are exposed to secondhand smoke in utero appear to be at risk for having a low birth weight. Children who are exposed to secondhand smoke are at an increased risk for respiratory problems and sudden infant death syndrome (SIDS).

THE BOTTOM LINE: Secondhand smoke is potentially dangerous to the baby and should be avoided when possible.

Selenium

Selenium is an antioxidant that is produced by the body. It is thought that selenium helps to repair damaged cells. Selenium can also be found in a variety of foods, including broccoli, cabbage, celery, cucumbers, garlic, mushrooms, organ meats, chicken, whole-grain products, egg yolks, and seafood.

CONCERNS: A recent study showed an association between lower selenium levels and miscarriage. However, more research needs to be done before selenium supplementation is recommended in pregnancy.

Selenium can be toxic if taken in large quantities. Doses over 700 to 1,100 micrograms are not recommended. Currently, there is no recommended daily allowance (RDA) for selenium. Since selenium supplements are categorized as food supplements, they are not regulated by the U.S. Food and Drug Administration. Thus, there is no guarantee of the strength, purity, or safety of these products. You should inform your health care provider if you are taking any nutritional supplements.

THE BOTTOM LINE: Until more research is done, it is not clear if supplementation with selenium will benefit women at risk for miscarriage. Supplementation should be avoided until more is known about selenium's effects during pregnancy and an RDA is established.

Sex

Sex includes sexual intercourse, oral sex, and other forms of sexual gratification.

CONCERNS: If you are having a pregnancy complication, you may be advised to abstain from sexual intercourse during your pregnancy. Examples of complications would be preterm labor, preterm contractions, premature rupture of membranes (PROM), and placenta previa (placenta covering your cervix).

Caution should be taken during oral sex so that no air is blown into a woman's vagina, which can theoretically increase the risk of an air embolism.

THE BOTTOM LINE: Sexual intercourse is safe throughout pregnancy unless you are having a pregnancy complication.

Shellfish ⚠

Shellfish are aquatic animals that have a shell of some kind. Popular shellfish include shrimp, clams, oysters, mussels, crab, scallops, and lobster.

CONCERNS: Certain varieties of shellfish may put you at risk for exposure to hepatitis A, the Norwalk virus, and the bacteria *Vibrio parahaemolyticus* and *Vibrio vulnificus*. These viruses and bacteria are responsible for many cases of food poisoning. Hepatitis A can be found in shellfish harvested in contaminated waters. Vaccination against hepatitis A is available and recommended to international travelers. The vaccination is theoretically safe in pregnancy but not routinely recommended. Thorough cooking of shellfish will adequately destroy hepatitis A, the Norwalk virus, and *Vibrio parahaemolyticus* and *Vibrio vulnificus*. *Campylobacter* (*see Campylobacter*) bacteria can also contaminate raw shellfish.

Bivalve mollusks (mussels, clams, oysters, and scallops) can also contain toxins that are produced by the algae that they consume. These toxins are heat and acid stable, meaning that they are not destroyed even when cooked. These toxins are more prevalent during the summer months when algae are more plentiful.

According to the U.S. Food and Drug Administration, raw shellfish, such as clams, oysters, and mussels, are the riskiest seafood and are responsible for many cases of food poisoning. However, the risks from raw shellfish appear to be lower than those from undercooked contaminated chicken. Keep in mind that these dangers are not increased during pregnancy and also exist when you are not pregnant.

Although many species of fish are now contaminated with mercury (*see* Methylmercury; Fish; Tuna), most shellfish appears to be low in mercury.

THE BOTTOM LINE: There is some risk of acquiring disease from shellfish, and cooking does not appear to completely eliminate that risk. You are not more susceptible to the risk because of pregnancy. You should avoid eating bivalves, especially during the warmer months.

Silica *See* Talcum powder.

Simethicone

Simethicone, also known as antigas medication, is sold under the brand names of Gas Relief®, Gas-X®, Mylanta®, Mylicon®, and Phazyme®. These over-the-counter medications act to break up gas bubbles in the digestive tract.

CONCERNS: It is thought that simethicone is not absorbed from the gastrointestinal tract and therefore should not cause any harm during pregnancy. Despite this, it is assigned a risk factor category of C (*see* Appendix 1) because not much is known about its effects.

THE BOTTOM LINE: Simethicone appears to be safe in pregnancy.

Skiing

Snow skiing is a form of exercise (*see* Exercise) that involves sliding down a mountain on skis in the snow. Water skiing involves being towed on skis behind a motor boat.

CONCERNS: Concerns about skiing and other sports center around the risk of falling during pregnancy. Most physicians recommend that you abstain from activities that have a high risk of falling during pregnancy because of an increased risk of placental abruption (premature separation of the placenta from the uterine wall).

Snow skiing also involves being at a higher altitude (*see* High altitude). Pregnancy at high altitude has been associated with low-birthweight babies, preeclampsia (hypertension, protein in the urine, and swelling), and preterm labor. High altitude also puts you at risk for altitude sickness. If you are visiting an area that has a high altitude, be aware of the symptoms of altitude sickness. These symptoms include insomnia, fatigue, headache, nausea, and vomiting. Try to keep well hydrated and limit activity if you feel dizzy or are short of breath.

THE BOTTOM LINE: Skiing is not recommended after the first trimester due to the risk of falling and causing injury. Abdominal trauma can lead to a placental abruption that can be dangerous to both mom and baby. Short visits to areas of high altitude are safe if you are having a healthy pregnancy, but please be sure to keep hydrated and look for signs of problems. Don't forget to use sunscreen, as your skin may be more sensitive to the effects of the sun during pregnancy (*see* Sun exposure).

Smoked fish ⚠️

Smoking is a process used to preserve food. There are several methods of smoking, including cold-smoking and hot-smoking. As a result, the food is only partially cooked. Smoked fish are often found in the refrigerated section of supermarkets and are commonly called nova style, lox, kippered, or jerky. Commonly smoked fish include salmon, whitefish, trout, cod, tuna, and mackerel.

CONCERNS: Because smoked fish are only partially cooked, they may be contaminated with *Listeria* (*see Listeria*). Pregnant women are 20 times more likely to get Listeriosis than other adults. Infected pregnant women may have symptoms similar to the flu, like fever and muscle aches, and infection may lead to preterm labor and stillbirth.

Concern over mercury (*see* Methylmercury) levels and other toxins in certain species of fish has motivated the Environmental Protection Agency (EPA) and the Food and Drug Administration (FDA) to release guidelines on fish consumption for pregnant women and young children. Tuna, shark, swordfish, king mackerel, and tile fish (a.k.a. golden or white snapper) are known to have higher levels of methylmercury. Fish that are low in mercury include salmon, cod, pollock, catfish, shrimp, and flounder. The Food and Drug Administration (FDA) recommends limiting fish high in mercury to two 6-ounce servings per week.

Other notable fish that should be limited during pregnancy, due to concerns over pollutants, are freshwater fish caught in local waters, as they are rarely monitored by the EPA. Polychlorinated biphenyls (PCBs) have been associated with decreased attention, memory, and IQ. Bluefish, striped bass, salmon, pike, trout, and walleye from contaminated lakes and rivers may contain PCBs within their fat. Check with your local health department to see if the fish in your area are known to be polluted.

THE BOTTOM LINE: Smoked fish such as salmon, whitefish, trout, cod, tuna, and mackerel should not be eaten unless cooked, canned, or labeled as "shelf-stable." Follow the FDA's recommendations on fish consumption to limit your intake of methylmercury and avoid locally caught fish not monitored by the EPA.

Smoking ⊘

Smoking refers to the smoking of tobacco products that generally contain nicotine (*see* Nicotine) and other dangerous chemicals. It has been estimated that 15 to 29 percent of pregnant women smoke tobacco during their pregnancies.

CONCERNS: Smoking has been clearly associated with several pregnancy complications, including ectopic pregnancy (pregnancy outside of the uterus), miscarriage, low birth weight, premature rupture of membranes, placenta previa (placenta covering the cervix), and placental abruption (premature separation of the placenta from the uterine wall). Smoking has also been associated with an increased incidence in sudden infant death syndrome (SIDS).

One recent study of pregnant women who smoked 10 or more cigarettes per day found increased numbers of chromosomal defects in the amniotic fluid cells. Chromosomal defects may lead to cancers in offspring.

THE BOTTOM LINE: Smoking tobacco has been associated with several serious pregnancy complications. Smoking should be avoided during your pregnancy. Ask your health care provider for help in quitting.

Sodium ☑

Sodium, more commonly referred to as salt, is required to maintain health. Your sodium requirements increase during pregnancy from 2,000 to 8,000 milligrams per day.

CONCERNS: In the past, pregnant women were advised to restrict their intake of sodium, as it was thought to contribute to swelling, increased blood pressure, and weight gain. However, this practice was not found to be beneficial, as a decrease in dietary sodium was associated with a decrease in overall diet quality. It is now thought that sodium should be consumed in moderation.

THE BOTTOM LINE: You may add salt to foods for taste in moderation. It is probably wise to limit the intake of processed foods, as these foods are generally high in sodium.

Soft cheeses ⚠️

Soft cheeses are made from cow, sheep, buffalo, or goat's milk. Some cheeses are pasteurized, a process in which dairy products are heated to kill harmful bacteria, while some are not. Soft cheeses are uncooked and have a high sugar and moisture content.

CONCERNS: Unpasteurized cheese (*see* Unpasteurized cheese; Cheese) may contain bacteria that are potentially harmful. These bacteria include *Listeria monocytogenes* (*see* Listeria), which can cause listeriosis, a flu-like illness characterized by fever, chills, and muscle aches. Pregnant women are 20 times more likely to get listeriosis than other healthy adults. Infection during pregnancy may lead to preterm labor and even stillbirth. All cheese made in the United States is made only from pasteurized milk. The Food and Drug Administration allows the importation of raw-milk cheese into the United States only if the cheese is aged 60 days or more. The harmful bacteria die as a result of the aging process. Young cheese aged less than 60 days made from unpasteurized milk is not allowed into the country.

Even if the cheese you are eating is made from pasteurized milk, contamination of soft cheese can occur. The Centers for Disease Control and Prevention (CDC) recommends avoiding all soft cheese, including blue-veined cheeses (*see* Blue-veined cheese), Brie (*see* Brie), camembert (*see* Camembert), feta (*see* Feta), and Mexican-style cheeses (*see* Mexican-style cheese) during pregnancy. Fresh mozzarella is also considered to be a soft cheese.

THE BOTTOM LINE: Unless cooked until bubbling, soft cheese should be avoided during pregnancy.

Sonograms ☑️

Sonograms, a.k.a. ultrasounds, use low-energy high-frequency sound waves to get images of the fetus. The sound waves bounce off the fetus, are detected by the emitting transducer, and are then displayed on a cathode ray tube.

CONCERNS: Although sonograms have been used for over 40 years, there is always some concern when a technology is used frequently and for long periods of time, especially when used on the unborn.

Most studies of ultrasound on pregnancy have shown no effects at all. However, a study of ultrasound use during pregnancy in monkeys showed an association with decreased birth weights, low white blood cell counts, and decreased muscle tone. A study in rats showed an association with slower learning rates the longer ultrasound was used. No study in human pregnancy has ever showed any association between ultrasound use and learning abnormalities.

Recently it has become possible to obtain a sonogram for the sole purpose of getting a picture of your baby. These sonograms are not ordered by physicians. There has been some controversy regarding this procedure in the medical community. Some of this concern focuses on the safety of repeated ultrasounds while other concern focuses on the possibility of a missed diagnosis as the person performing the ultrasound may not be trained to pick up an abnormality. The American Pregnancy Association recommends that women obtain sonograms from licensed medically trained practitioners.

THE BOTTOM LINE: Sonograms ordered by a physician are considered to be safe in pregnancy.

Soy

The term *soy* refers to many products that are made from soybeans. Soybeans are rich in calcium, iron, B vitamins, zinc, and protein.

CONCERNS: Soybeans have been found to contain isoflavones, a class of phytoestrogens that are plant-derived compounds with some estrogenic effects. Pregnant laboratory rats who consumed diets rich in soy had pups that showed evidence of increased masculinization. However, these rats were fed extremely high doses of phytoestrogens. There is no evidence that moderate amounts of soy products in your diet can cause harm to a developing fetus.

THE BOTTOM LINE: Soy in moderation is considered to be safe and beneficial in pregnancy. Higher doses of dietary soy are still being investigated.

Spas ⚠

The term *spas* refers to both hot tubs and places that offer treatments, such as massage, facials, and skin exfoliation.

CONCERNS: Numerous studies have shown an association between elevated temperatures and the increased incidence of neural tube defects and miscarriages. Hot tubs (*see* Hot tubs) appear to be dangerous if your core body temperature (CBT) rises to 102.5°F/39°C. Some researchers have suggested that if a pregnant woman's CBT becomes that high, she would feel uncomfortable and get out of the tub.

A recent study found that pregnant women who received a massage (*see* Massage) two times per week for five weeks had better sleep patterns, lower anxiety levels, less back pain, and lower levels of stress hormones. Other studies have shown an association between prenatal massage and decreased preterm labor and neonatal problems. Massage is also known to reduce the pain during labor.

Noninvasive facials and skin treatments have not been associated with pregnancy complications. Use caution when considering "mini facelifts" and Botox® treatments (*see* Botox; Glycolic peels).

THE BOTTOM LINE: Taking a bath in water below 100°F/38°C is considered to be safe during pregnancy. If you don't have a thermometer handy, dip your elbow or forearm into the water. If the water is a comfortable temperature, it is probably safe. If your skin becomes red or you notice that you are sweating, the water is probably too hot. For a masseur, look for a referral from the American Massage Therapy Association and ask if they have any experience with prenatal massage. Facials and noninvasive skin treatments are considered to be safe during pregnancy.

Speed Stack® ⚠

Speed Stack® is a brand name of an energy drink (*see* Energy drinks).

Splenda®

Splenda® is a brand name of an artificial sweetener (*see* Sucralose).

Sprouts, raw

Raw sprouts can be found in the produce section of food markets and in salads. They are the sprouts from germinated beans and seeds. There are many varieties, but a few of the more common ones include alfalfa sprouts, mung bean sprouts, and lentil sprouts. Unless canned, sprouts should be kept refrigerated. Sprouts can be grown at home easily.

CONCERNS: Raw sprouts have been linked to contamination with the bacteria *Escherichia coli* (*see* E. coli infection). *E. coli* can cause bloody diarrhea and abdominal cramps, and some strains have been known to cause death. *Salmonella* (*see* Salmonella) has also been known to contaminate raw alfalfa sprouts. Infection with *Salmonella* while pregnant has been associated with miscarriage, preterm labor, and stillbirth.

THE BOTTOM LINE: Raw sprouts can be contaminated with harmful bacteria. Cooking sprouts will ensure their safety.

Stress

According to the American College of Obstetrics and Gynecology, stress is defined as any real or perceived trauma, whether physical or psychological, that results in the release of stress hormones.

CONCERNS: Studies have shown that women who experience stress during their pregnancy are more likely to have low-birth-weight babies and preterm labor. However, a recent meta-analytic review was conducted using previous studies done on the relationship between maternal anxiety and adverse fetal outcomes. This review failed to show any association between anxiety and adverse pregnancy outcomes.

THE BOTTOM LINE: Although we all experience stress in our lives, do what you can to relieve this stress. If you feel anxious or believe that you have significant stress, discuss this with your health care provider and consider therapy.

Sucralose ☑

Sucralose, also known as Splenda®, is an artificial sweetener (*see* Artificial sweeteners). It is found in many diet drinks and diet foods as well as baked goods, salad dressings, jams and jellies, and chewing gum.

CONCERNS: Sucralose is one of the newest artificial sweeteners available. It is produced by substituting three chlorine atoms for three hydrogen-oxygen groups on regular sugar, so it passes through the body without being metabolized.

One recent study examining the effects of sucralose on pregnant rats and rabbits failed to show any teratogenic (cause of birth defects) effects on offspring.

THE BOTTOM LINE: The U.S. Food and Drug Administration has determined sucralose to be a safe additive even during pregnancy. However, it is a new product and no long-term studies are available. Until more is known, it seems wise to limit your intake during pregnancy.

Sun exposure ⚠

Exposure to the sun causes exposure to ultraviolet B (UVB) rays. UVB rays tend to be more intense between 10 A.M. and 4 P.M., during the summer months, at high altitudes, and along the equator.

CONCERNS: UVB radiation does not penetrate farther than the skin and will not reach the fetus. UVB has not been shown to be dangerous to a developing pregnancy. However, frequent exposure to sun can cause skin wrinkling, premature aging, and skin cancer.

During pregnancy, skin can become more sensitive to the effects of the sun, possibly due to increased hormonal levels. Some women tend to burn more easily. Other women can develop chloasma (the mask of pregnancy), a facial discoloration on the forehead, nose, and cheeks. Sun exposure can make this condition more noticeable.

Some sunscreens have been associated with allergic reactions. Studies in animals have not found any of the active ingredients in sunscreens to be teratogenic (causing birth defects), but studies have not been performed on humans.

THE BOTTOM LINE: As when not pregnant, continue to use a daily sunscreen and try to avoid exposure when UVB rays are most intense.

⚠

Sushi

Sushi is a Japanese food based on boiled rice flavored with sweetened vinegar. Raw fish and vegetables are then added to the rice.

CONCERNS: Sushi is of concern due to the use of raw fish. Raw fish can become contaminated with the bacteria *Listeria* (*see Listeria*) Pregnant women are 20 times more likely to get listeriosis than other healthy adults. Infected pregnant women may have symptoms similar to the flu, like fever and muscle aches, and infection may lead to preterm labor and even stillbirth.

Raw fish may also contain parasites, like the tapeworm. Freezing the fish prior to consumption, which is often done for sushi, will kill adult parasitic worms, but small eggs in the flesh of the fish may persist.

Certain varieties of shellfish (*see* Shellfish) may put you at risk for exposure to hepatitis A, the Norwalk virus, and the bacteria *Vibrio parahaemolyticus, Vibrio vulnificus* and *Campylobacter* (*see Campylobacter*). These viruses and bacteria are responsible for many cases of food poisoning. Hepatitis A can be found in shellfish harvested in contaminated waters. Vaccination against hepatitis A is available and recommended to international travelers. The vaccination is theoretically safe in pregnancy but not routinely recommended. Thorough cooking of shellfish will adequately destroy hepatitis A, the Norwalk virus and *Vibrio parahaemolyticus, Vibrio vulnificus*, and *Campylobacter*.

Recently, the U.S. Food and Drug Administration (FDA) has voiced concern over the methylmercury (*see* Methylmercury) levels in many commonly consumed fish. When consumed in high doses, methylmercury is known to be harmful to a baby's developing neurologic system. The FDA has recommended safe amounts of different varieties of fish for pregnant women and young children. Keep in mind that these recommendations may change with the health of our ecosystems. Tuna (*see* Tuna), shark, swordfish, king mackerel, and tile fish (a.k.a. golden or white snapper) are known to contain high levels of methylmercury. Fish that are low in mercury and are considered to be safe include salmon, cod, pollock, catfish, shrimp, and flounder.

THE BOTTOM LINE: Eating raw fish does put you at risk for food poisoning and parasites. If you are concerned, stick to sushi made with only vegetables or cooked fish. The FDA inspects and labels seafood harvested from safe areas as such. By going to a busy, reputable sushi restaurant, you can limit your risk of buying contaminated seafood. Fish is a good source of protein and omega-3 fatty acids.

Swimming ⚠️

Swimming is an excellent form of exercise (*see* Exercise) during pregnancy because it is low impact and keeps your core body temperature low. The American College of Obstetrics and Gynecology recommends 30 minutes of exercise per day on most days of pregnancy.

CONCERNS: Swimming pools are often treated with several chemicals, including chlorine (*see* Chlorine), to destroy bacteria. A few studies have found that a group of by-products of chlorine, trihalomethanes (THMs), can be found in water treated with chlorine and is associated with low birth weight and fetal birth defects, such as neural tube defects. THMs can be absorbed through the skin and lungs. It is unclear what levels are dangerous during pregnancy. Other studies have not found this association. Chlorine can also break down to chloroform, which may also cause harm during a pregnancy. The Environmental Protection Agency (EPA) has set up standards to monitor these levels and is continuing to do research on this issue.

Swimming outdoors puts you at risk for sun exposure (*see* Sun exposure) and care should be taken to use sunscreen.

Finally, there is always the possibility that untreated water can contain harmful bacteria. *E. coli* (*see E. coli* infection) can sometimes contaminate lake water and certain strains can cause infection.

THE BOTTOM LINE: Swimming is an excellent form of exercise during pregnancy. Until more is known about the chemicals used in pool water, we must depend on the EPA to ensure our safety. If newer research confirms the reports of increased birth defects from swimming in water with high THMs, stricter standards and testing will need to be implemented. THM levels have been shown to be higher in pool water during busy use, so try to swim when the pool is less crowded. Outdoor pools and pools with high ceilings may have lower levels of THMs in the air and may be a safer option. Rinse off any chemicals after you leave the pool. Use sunscreen if swimming outside. Try to avoid swallowing lake water.

Swimming pool *See* Pools.

Talcum powder ⚠️

Talcum powder is a powder made from zinc stearate and magnesium silicates. It is frequently used to prevent and treat diaper rash.

CONCERNS: The ingredients of the powder are finely ground and can easily be inhaled to cause respiratory problems. Due to this, talcum powder has fallen out of favor among the medical community.

Talcum powder use in the female genital area has been associated with an increased incidence of cervical cancer, although this association has not clearly been proven.

THE BOTTOM LINE: It is unclear whether talcum powder can cause harm. However, dermatologists have not found any advantage to using powders over ointments in treating diaper rash. To avoid inhalation and possible respiratory problems, it is probably wise to switch to using an ointment or powder made from cornstarch.

Tamiflu® ⚠️

Tamiflu® (oseltamivir phosphate) is a medication taken in the form of a capsule or liquid that is used to prevent or treat influenza caused by the influenza virus types A and B (see Appendix 3).

CONCERNS: There are a few case reports of pregnant women who have been prescribed Tamiflu® and have had no adverse pregnancy effects. Tamiflu® has been assigned a pregnancy risk factor category of C (see Appendix 1).

THE BOTTOM LINE: Until more data is available, Tamiflu® is not routinely recommended during pregnancy. Tamiflu® should not replace routine immunization (*see* Immunizations).

Tanning beds

Tanning beds generally emit ultraviolet A (UVA) radiation to result in tanning.

CONCERNS: Radiation in high doses is known to cause birth defects. However, UVA radiation does not penetrate farther than the skin and will not reach the fetus. UVA radiation has not been shown to be dangerous to a developing pregnancy. However, frequent exposure to sun can cause skin wrinkling, premature aging, and skin cancer.

Tanning beds emit two to five times more UVA rays than natural sunlight. The skin of pregnant women may be more sensitive to the sun (*see* Sun exposure) and to UV rays. Studies show that women who routinely use tanning beds have an increased incidence of melanoma (a type of skin cancer).

Finally, if your core body temperature rises above 102°F/39°C during tanning bed use during the first trimester, you may have an increased risk of having a baby born with a neural tube defect.

THE BOTTOM LINE: Although tanning beds have not been shown to cause any harm to the baby, use caution, as your skin may be more sensitive during pregnancy.

Tanning sprays and creams

Tanning sprays and creams are used to create the appearance of a tan. The active ingredient in self-tanners is dihydroxyacetone (DHA).

CONCERNS: Tanning sprays and creams are applied to the surface of the skin. Little is known about how much, if any, is absorbed into the skin. There have been no reported adverse effects due to self-tanners during pregnancy, but information is limited.

THE BOTTOM LINE: Tanning creams and lotions appear to be safe during pregnancy. If you crave a tan, using self-tanners is probably safer than using tanning beds or lying out in the sun.

Tap water

⚠

Tap water is the water that you can get directly from your sink. Tap water may contain a variety of chemicals. Some are purposefully added, while others are added inadvertently as a result of contamination.

CONCERNS: To ensure the safety of our water supply, water is treated with a variety of chemicals to destroy potential pathogens. The Environmental Protection Agency (EPA) regulates the chemicals found in drinking water through testing, reporting, and public notification. Recent reports have found that women who drank tap water during pregnancy had more children with birth defects and miscarriages than those who drank bottled water. However, keep in mind that these types of studies are often difficult to assess, as the women were exposed to many different chemicals and pollutants. A list of some of the chemicals added to and found in our drinking water follows.

- *Chlorine* (*see* Chlorine): A few studies have found that a by-product of chlorine, trihalomethane (THM), can be found in water treated with chlorine and is associated with low birth weight and fetal birth defects, such as neural tube defects. Other studies have not found this association. THM can be absorbed by drinking or through the skin and lungs. It is unclear what levels are dangerous during pregnancy. Chlorine can also break down into chloroform, which may also cause harm during pregnancy. The EPA has set up standards to monitor these levels and is continuing to do research on this issue.

- *Sodium fluoride* (*see* Fluoride): There is an established government recommended daily allowance for fluoride, and the element is known to be toxic in high quantities. Studies have shown that fluoride can cross the placenta, and since 1966 the U.S. Food and Drug Administration has banned the use of advertising and labeling of fluoride supplements for prenatal use. One study has demonstrated a link between fluoride supplementation and attention deficit hyperactivity disorder (ADHD) in children. Other researchers have claimed that fluoride supplementation could help reduce the risk of birth defects, including neural tube defects. Some studies have reported that fluoride supplementation is completely safe during pregnancy.

- *Lead (see* Lead): Exposure to high levels of lead has been associated with spontaneous abortion, preterm labor, and premature rupture of membranes. Lead has never been linked to any major congenital abnormalities, but some studies have found a variety of minor malformations associated with high lead levels. Prenatal exposure to lead has also been associated with lower mental development scores in infants. Studies using laboratory rats have concluded that lead in their drinking water may be responsible for the development of chronic diseases, such as asthma (*see* Asthma), cancer, and allergies.

- *Pesticides, herbicides, and fertilizer (see* Pesticides; Herbicides; Fertilizer): Pesticides and herbicides have been associated with intrauterine growth restriction (low birth weight), birth defects, and developmental abnormalities.

THE BOTTOM LINE: We must depend on the EPA to ensure the safety of our drinking water. Well water is not monitored by the EPA. If you are concerned about substances in your drinking water, contact the EPA for more information, consider drinking bottled water or using a filter, and have your water tested.

Tattoos

A tattoo involves placing ink under the skin to create a permanent skin decoration.

CONCERNS: There are several concerns about tattoos including possible infection (HIV, Hepatitis B and C) from contaminated needles, initiating labor, differences in skin during pregnancy, the safety of ink pigments, and fainting.

The most serious concern is the risk of infection. However, with proper technique this risk is markedly reduced. No scientific studies have been done specifically examining an increased risk of preterm labor or the teratogenicity of pigments used and there are no case reports suggesting that these concerns are reasonable.

While most anesthesiologists will place an epidural on a woman with a back tattoo, some women with back tattoos have been inaccurately told that they would not be able to get an epidural for labor analgesia/anesthesia. If you are concerned, consult the policies of your hospital.

THE BOTTOM LINE: Although tattoos are probably safe, there are no scientific studies examining the risk of getting tattoos during pregnancy. If you are concerned about acquiring an infection, wait to get a tattoo until after your delivery.

Taurine ⚠️

Taurine is a nonessential amino acid. It is found in meat, dairy, and seafood and may be added to many energy drinks (see Energy drinks). Its best established use is in the treatment of congestive heart failure. There is no recommended daily allowance, as it can be formed by the body from Vitamin B_6 (see Vitamin B_6) and other amino acids.

CONCERNS: Because taurine is categorized as a food supplement, it is not regulated by the U.S. Food and Drug Administration. Thus, there is no guarantee of the strength, purity, or safety of this product. You should inform your health care provider if you are taking any nutritional supplements.

THE BOTTOM LINE: Because taurine is an amino acid, it is generally considered to be safe. Maximum safe doses for pregnant women have not been established, and supplementation should be avoided during pregnancy.

Tea ⚠️

Tea is made from an infusion of tea leaves (also known as the *Camellia sinensis* plant). Tea can be further classified into black, green, Oolong, red, or white tea. These distinctions are based on the way the tea leaves are processed. Black tea leaves are fermented before being heated and dried and make a dark reddish brown brew. Green tea is produced from leaves that are steamed and then dried, and they produce a yellow greenish tea. Oolong tea is partially fermented and then heated and dried to produce a tea that is in between black and green. Red tea is fully fermented and is synonymous with black tea. White tea leaves are picked before the leaves are fully opened, and the tea is similar to green tea in that it is not fermented. Teas may contain caffeine or may be decaffeinated. Black and red tea have the most caffeine while white and green teas have the lowest amounts of caffeine. Herb tea (see Herb tea) is made from an infusion of a variety of herbs, flowers, and spices and does not contain caffeine.

CONCERNS: It is well known that caffeine (see Caffeine) can stimulate the central nervous system, kidneys, and heart and cause the release of insulin from the pancreas. In 1980 the Food and Drug Administration (FDA) cautioned women against caffeine use during pregnancy based on animal studies. However, since that time the FDA has amended its initial warning based on research that indicated that moderate caffeine use does not appear to cause birth defects. Some studies have shown that high amounts of caffeine during pregnancy are associated with intrauterine growth restriction (low birth weight). In light of this, most health care providers suggest a reduction in caffeine during pregnancy. If less than 300 mg is consumed per day, there appears to be little risk. The difficulty lies in calculating that amount since caffeine amounts differ from cup to cup. The amount of caffeine in tea ranges from 20 to 110 milligrams per 8-ounce serving.

Green tea has been gaining in popularity in the United States due to some recent studies that have suggested that the high levels of antioxidants in green tea may be beneficial in the prevention of cancer, heart disease, and inflammatory conditions. Similarly, white tea is also thought to have high levels of antioxidants. Another study has also found that a compound found in green tea may stop the growth of cancer cells. While this is an exciting finding, the same compound can interfere with folic acid (see Folic acid), a vitamin that has been shown to decrease the risk of neural tube defects.

Another concern centers on the fact that some teas make it more difficult to absorb iron (*see* Iron).

Some herb teas may also be of some concern as herbs are often used as medicinal remedies and can have clear physiological effects. However, there has been very little research done on the safety of herbal teas during pregnancy and they are not regulated as drugs by the FDA.

Many herbal tea mixtures are sold as "pregnancy" teas to promote uterine and pregnancy health. Examples of herbal teas recommended during pregnancy include camomile (*see* Camomile tea), cinnamon, dandelion, lavender, lemon balm, nettle, red raspberry, rose hips, spearmint, stevia, and wild oats. Some herbal teas are used to induce labor. They include anise, beth root, black cohosh, blue cohosh, borage, cramp bark, dill, lobelia, nettle, spikenard, red raspberry, and squaw vine. Use caution with these teas prior to term.

According to the FDA, commercially prepared teas in moderate amounts appear to be safe. If the ingredients are considered to be safe as foods (cinnamon, citrus peel, mint, ginger, lemon balm, and rose hip), they are considered to be safe in teas.

THE BOTTOM LINE: Three hundred milligrams or less of caffeine per day is safe during pregnancy. High amounts of green tea may interfere with folic acid, so limit intake until more information is available. Use caution when consuming herbal teas because little is known about their safety during pregnancy.

Teeth-bleaching

Teeth-bleaching is a procedure that uses chemicals to whiten teeth. This procedure can be performed at a dentist's office or at home. The most common bleaching gel is carbamide peroxide, whose active ingredient is hydrogen peroxide.

CONCERNS: As this is a relatively new procedure, not much is known about the safety of teeth-bleaching during pregnancy. Some dentists will do it while others will suggest waiting until after pregnancy. So far no bad effects have been reported. Although you swallow some of the whitening material, it is unlikely that much is absorbed.

A second issue is that some women find that the whitening agents affect their gums. The increase in gum sensitivity caused by pregnancy may make the procedure uncomfortable.

The U.S. Food and Drug Administration does not recognize teeth-bleaching products as drugs and does not regulate them.

THE BOTTOM LINE: Teeth whiteners are probably safe during pregnancy. Until we have more information about their effects during pregnancy, many dentists recommend waiting.

Terazole®

Terazole® is the brand name for terconazole (*see* Terconazole; Antifungal medications, oral and topical).

Terconazole

Terconazole is an antifungal medication (*see* Antifungal medications, oral and topical) available under the brand name Terazole®. Terconazole is used to treat fungal infections, such as yeast infections.

CONCERNS: Terconazole has not been associated with any adverse pregnancy outcomes. Terconazole has been assigned a risk factor category of C (*see* Appendix 1).

THE BOTTOM LINE: Terconazole is considered to be safe in pregnancy.

Tetracycline

Tetracycline is an antibiotic (*see* Antibiotics, oral) that can be taken either orally or intravenously.

CONCERNS: Use of tertracycline during pregnancy can cause staining of the fetal teeth. This occurs due to an interaction between tetracycline and calcium as the teeth are forming in utero. Tetracycline has been assigned a risk factor category of D and should not be taken during pregnancy.

THE BOTTOM LINE: Tetracycline should not be taken during pregnancy.

Thiamine ☑

Thiamine, also known as Vitamin B₁, is a water-soluble B complex vitamin. It is thought to play a role in carbohydrate metabolism. It can be found in fortified breads, cereals, pasta, whole grains, lean meats, fish, dried beans, peas, soybeans, and multivitamins (*see* Multivitamins). The recommended daily allowance (RDA) during pregnancy is 1.5 milligrams.

CONCERNS: There are a few reports of women taking large doses of thiamine during pregnancy that resulted in babies having neurologic problems. Thiamine has a risk factor category of A if used in recommended doses and a risk factor category of C if used in higher doses (*see* Appendix 1).

THE BOTTOM LINE: The RDA of thiamine is safe during pregnancy. Large doses should be avoided.

Tick collars *See* Flea and tick medication. ⚠

Toxoplasmosis ⚠

Toxoplasmosis is an illness caused by a parasite called *Toxoplasmosis gondii*. Symptoms of this illness include fever, enlarged and tender lymph nodes, fatigue, sore throat, and a rash. Often there are no symptoms at all. *Toxoplasmosis* is a common childhood infection, and many adults are immune. This parasite can enter a cat (*see* Cats; Litter boxes) when it eats raw meat (usually birds) and then is passed through its feces. The cat owner can then acquire the parasite via hand-to-mouth contact after touching the contaminated feces. It is much more common to get *Toxoplasmosis* from eating raw or undercooked meat (*see* Cured meat; Deli meats, cooked and uncooked), from soil that has been visited by infected cats (*see* Gardening), and from unwashed vegetables.

CONCERNS: *Toxoplasmosis* can cause fetal death, preterm labor, and some kinds of birth defects. Many people are immune to it, and a quick blood test from your health care provider will reveal whether you are immune.

THE BOTTOM LINE: Wash hands carefully after changing cat litter, or, better yet, have someone else do this chore; wear gloves when gardening; cook your meat well; and wash all vegetables, cutting boards, and utensils carefully.

Trampolines ⚠️

Trampolines are a piece of exercise equipment that allows you to jump and flip.

CONCERNS: Concern about many sports during pregnancy centers on the risk of falling. Most physicians recommend that you abstain from exercise (*see* Exercise) that has a high risk of falling during pregnancy because of an increased risk of placental abruption (premature separation of the placenta from the uterine wall). Using a trampoline would certainly put you at risk for losing your balance and falling on your abdomen.

THE BOTTOM LINE: Although there are no studies evaluating the use of trampolines during pregnancy, it would seem wise to avoid this exercise during pregnancy.

Tretinoin ⚠️

Tretinoin, sold under the brand name Retin-A®, is a cream that is used in the treatment of acne and other skin problems. Tretinoin's active ingredient is a retinoid and a relative of vitamin A (*see* Vitamin A).

CONCERNS: Since Accutane® (*see* Isotretinoin), which is known to cause birth defects, and Retin-A® are both retinoids, there has been some concern over the use of Retin-A® creams during pregnancy. However, it has been estimated that less than 10 percent of the Retin-A® passes into the mother's bloodstream following topical use. So far, no known adverse pregnancy outcomes have been associated with Retin-A® use during pregnancy.

Retin-A® stays in the body approximately one week after use. If you are concerned about any potential effects, it is recommended that you stop using this product for more than one week prior to becoming pregnant.

Tretinoin has been assigned a risk factor category of C (*see* Appendix 1).

THE BOTTOM LINE: Until more is known, it is probably best to limit or avoid Retin-A® cream during pregnancy. However, no clear reports indicate that there is a danger to using this topical product during pregnancy.

Triamcinolone acetonide

Triamcinolone acetonide is an antihistamine (*see* Allergy medications; Antihistamines). A brand name for this drug is Nasacort®.

CONCERNS: Triamcinolone acetonide has been assigned a risk factor category of C in the second and third trimesters and a risk factor category of D in the first trimester (*see* Appendix 1).

THE BOTTOM LINE: Triamcinolone acetonide is safe to take during pregnancy after the first trimester.

Trichomoniasis

Trichomoniasis is caused by a parasite (*see* Parasites) called *Trichomonas vaginalis*. Vaginal infection with this organism can cause vaginal discharge, pain with urination, itching, burning, and odor. Trichomoniasis is diagnosed by looking at the vaginal discharge on a slide under a microscope. It is easily treated with the antibiotic metronidazole (*see* Antibiotics, oral; Metronidazole).

CONCERNS: Infection with *Trichomonas* during pregnancy has been associated with preterm labor and preterm rupture of membranes. It has not been associated with any birth defects.

THE BOTTOM LINE: Trichomoniasis is a common vaginal infection. It should be treated during pregnancy.

Tucks®

Tucks® is a brand name for a hemorrhoid medication (*see* Hemorrhoid medications).

Tums®

Tums® is a brand name for an antacid (*see* Antacids).

Tuna

Tuna is a commonly consumed fish (*see* Fish) that can be purchased raw or cooked and packed in a can or bag. Tuna is high in protein and essential fatty acids that help your baby's developing brain. Albacore tuna refers to white tuna or tuna steak. "Light" canned tuna is a mix of albacore tuna and darker tuna meat and actually has lower levels of mercury than pure albacore tuna.

CONCERNS: Tuna is a large predatory fish. Following ingestion of smaller fish contaminated with mercury, high amounts of mercury becomes stored in the cells of the tuna. Recently the U.S. Food and Drug Administration (FDA) has voiced concern over the mercury levels in many commonly consumed fish. When tuna is consumed in high doses, certain bacteria can convert naturally occurring and manmade mercury into methylmercury. Methylmercury can accumulate in the fatty tissue of certain fish. Methylmercury is known to be harmful to a baby's developing neurologic system. The FDA has recommended safe amounts of different varieties of fish for pregnant women and young children. Keep in mind that these recommendations may change with the health of our ecosystems.

THE BOTTOM LINE: The FDA recommends no more than two 6-ounce cans of tuna a week or 12 ounces of other cooked tuna per week (about two servings per week), if that is the only type of fish that you eat. If you are eating other types of fish, the amount of tuna you eat may need to be reduced.

Tylenol®

Tylenol® is a brand name for acetaminophen (*see* Acetaminophen; Pain relievers).

Ultrasounds *See* Sonograms. ✓

Underwire bras ✓

Underwire bras have a covered wire in the bra for added support.

CONCERNS: There have been some reports that underwire bras can put pressure on milk ducts and increase your risk of having a clogged milk duct. Although no scientific studies have looked specifically at this problem, it is likely that a well-fitting and comfortable bra, underwire or not, will not cause any problems during your pregnancy or while you are nursing.

THE BOTTOM LINE: If the bra is comfortable and does not cause any pain, it is probably well fitting and will not cause any pregnancy complications.

Unpasteurized cheeses ⚠

Unpasteurized cheeses (*see* Cheese) are made from unpasteurized milk. The pasteurization process involves cooking the milk to kill any harmful bacteria. Examples of cheese that can be made with unpasteurized milk include blue-veined cheeses (*see* Blue-veined cheese), Brie (*see* Brie), camembert (*see* Camembert cheese), feta (*see* Feta), and many Mexican-style cheeses (*see* Mexican-style cheese).

CONCERNS: Unpasteurized cheese may contain bacteria that are potentially harmful. These bacteria include *Listeria monocytogenes* (*see* Listeria), which can cause listeriosis, a flu-like illness characterized by fever, chills, and muscle aches. Pregnant women are 20 times more likely to get listeriosis than other healthy adults. Infection during pregnancy may lead to preterm labor and even stillbirth.

All cheese made in the United States is made only from pasteurized milk. The U.S. Food and Drug Administration allows the importation of raw-milk cheese into the United States only if the cheese is aged 60 days or more. The harmful bacteria die as a result of the aging process. Young cheese aged less than 60 days made from unpasteurized milk is not allowed into the country.

THE BOTTOM LINE: The Centers for Disease Control and Prevention recommends avoiding unpasteurized cheese during pregnancy. Use caution if traveling abroad.

Unpasteurized juice

Unpasteurized juice includes any juice that has not been cooked to kill any harmful bacteria. Such juices are commonly found in the refrigerated section of markets and at farm stands.

CONCERNS: Although the process of pasteurization kills harmful bacteria, it may also break down vitamins and nutrients. Ninety-eight percent of juice sold in this country is pasteurized. Unpasteurized juices may contain harmful bacteria, including *Escherichia coli* (*see E. coli* infection) and *Salmonella* (*see Salmonella*). These bacteria can be dangerous to people with weakened immune systems. As a result, the U.S. Food and Drug Administration requires unpasteurized juices to be labeled as such.

THE BOTTOM LINE: Avoid unpasteurized juice during pregnancy. If you are unsure, bring the juice to a boil before consuming it to kill any harmful bacteria.

Urinary tract infections

Urinary tract infections (UTIs) are infections of the bladder caused by bacteria. Symptoms include a burning sensation when you urinate, blood in the urine, and urinary frequency (having to urinate frequently).

CONCERNS: It may be easier to get a UTI while you are pregnant. This may be due to increased hormonal levels and the fact that the enlarging uterus puts pressure on the ureters (the tubes that connect the kidneys to the bladder). It has been estimated that 8 percent of pregnant women get a UTI. An untreated UTI can lead to development of a more serious condition called pyelonephritis (infection of the kidneys).

If you are diagnosed with a UTI, your health care provider will probably recommend that you take oral antibiotics (*see* Antibiotics) for 7 to 10 days.

THE BOTTOM LINE: Untreated UTIs during pregnancy are not only uncomfortable but may lead to more serious infections. UTIs are easily treated with antibiotics, many of which are considered safe in pregnancy.

Vaccines *See* Immunizations.

Valium®

Valium® is a brand name for diazepam (*see* Psychiatric medications).

Valorin®

Valorin® is a brand name for acetaminophen (*see* Acetaminophen; Pain relievers).

Vaporizers

Vaporizers are machines that humidify the air by vaporizing water. They may create cold-water vapor or may have a heating unit to warm the water to make warm vapor. Some people add medicines or essential oils to the water to be vaporized.

CONCERNS: As with air conditioners and humidifiers (*see* Air conditioners; Humidifiers), there has been some publicity about the association of Legionnaire's disease outbreaks with vaporizers. Legionnaire's disease is caused by a bacterium called *Legionella pneumophila*, which lives in warm-water environments such as those found in air conditioners, plumbing systems, and humidifiers. It is estimated that 8,000 to 10,000 people contract Legionnaire's disease every year. However, it is often difficult to diagnose the disease accurately because symptoms can vary from person to person. Unless a doctor specifically suspects Legionnaire's, the appropriate tests are often not performed. The disease is most dangerous to those who have a weakened immune system due to cancer therapy, smoking, or organ transplants. Pregnancy does not appear to be an increased risk factor for getting this disease. While the U.S. Department of Labor's Occupational Safety and Health Administration has standards in place for work-related systems, it is unclear how many cases of Legionnaire's disease are acquired in private homes and what the optimal methods of prevention are. Proper maintenance of all plumbing systems, air-conditioning systems, and humidifiers should minimize your risk of contracting this disease.

Vaporizers are also great places for mold to grow. Some people are allergic to mold, so your vaporizer should be properly cleaned and maintained. Follow the manufacturer's recommendations for proper maintenance.

THE BOTTOM LINE: A well-maintained vaporizer is safe in pregnancy and may be beneficial for reducing the discomfort of dry skin and nasal passageways.

Venom®

Venom® is a brand name of an energy drink (*see* Energy drinks).

Vicks® VapoRub®

Vicks® VapoRub® is a topical ointment used to treat cough and congestion from the common cold and muscle aches and pains. The active ingredients include camphor, eucalyptus oil, menthol, and turpentine oil. Inactive ingredients include cedar leaf oil and nutmeg oil.

CONCERNS: Although Vicks® VapoRub® has been used for many years without adverse pregnancy outcomes, there is minimal data on its safety during pregnancy. One study on camphor in laboratory rats and rabbits during pregnancy demonstrated that high doses caused convulsions and decreased food intake and reduced body weight gain and reduced food consumption. However, the camphor was administered orally and at high doses, and the study failed to show any fetal malformations.

Many of the oils in Vicks® VapoRub® may be considered essential oils (*see* Essential oils). Some practitioners who use essential oils suggest avoiding their use during pregnancy.

THE BOTTOM LINE: Vicks® VapoRub®, when used as directed, appears to be safe during pregnancy.

Vitamin A ⚠️

Vitamin A is a fat-soluble vitamin that is important for the development of fetal organs, including the eyes, heart, and limbs. Vitamin A can be found in two forms: preformed or retinoid, which originates from animal tissue and can be obtained through meat and dairy foods and from vitamin supplements and supplemented foods, and retinol, which is made in the body from beta-carotene (*see* Beta-carotene) and can be obtained from fruits, vegetable, and vitamin supplements.

CONCERNS: Preformed Vitamin A is considered to be a teratogen (causing birth defects) in high doses. However, the amount needed to cause birth defects is controversial. One study has shown that women who took 10,000 international units (3,000 RE) per day during pregnancy were five times more likely to have a child with a birth defect. The Tetrology Society has estimated that taking greater than 25,000 international units (7,500 RE) per day of preformed Vitamin A in pregnancy would cause one in 57 infants to have a birth defect.

There have been no studies showing that large amounts of beta-carotene lead to toxicity or birth defects. The Tetrology Society has concluded that beta-carotene is not a human teratogen. For this reason, beta-carotene is often added to multivitamins (*see* Multivitamins) to ensure adequate intake of Vitamin A without the risks of teratogenic effects.

The U.S. Food and Drug Administration has set the recommended daily allowance of preformed Vitamin A to be 8,000 international units (2,400 RE) per day during pregnancy. Vitamin A has been assigned a risk factor category A in normal doses and a risk factor category of X (*see* Appendix 1) in doses above the U.S. RDA.

Finally, consider that Accutane® (*see* Isotretinoin) and Retin-A® (*see* Tretinoin), prescription drugs used to treat severe acne, are synthetic forms of Vitamin A. Accutane® is known to cause birth defects and should be avoided during pregnancy. There are no clear reports on whether there is a danger to using Retin-A® cream during pregnancy.

THE BOTTOM LINE: It seems safe to take a maximum of 5,000 to 8,000 international units (1,500 to 2,900 RE) of preformed Vitamin A per day in pregnancy. Check your multivitamin ingredients; you should take one that does not exceed 5,000 international units (1,500 RE) of preformed Vitamin A per day, since you will get some preformed Vitamin A in your diet. Products that have Vitamin A as a food additive (*see* Food additives) should be labeled as such.

Vitamin B$_1$ *See* Thiamine.

Vitamin B$_2$ *See* Riboflavin.

Vitamin B$_3$ *See* Niacin.

Vitamin B$_6$ *See* Pyridoxine.

Vitamin B$_9$ *See* Folic acid.

Vitamin B$_{12}$

Vitamin B$_{12}$, or cyanocobalamin, is a water-soluble B complex vitamin important for cell reproduction, cell growth, and the formation of myelin. Vitamin B$_{12}$ can be found in meat, eggs, and dairy products. The recommended daily allowance (RDA) in pregnancy is 2.2 micrograms.

CONCERNS: Women who are strict vegetarians who do not eat any dairy often take Vitamin B$_{12}$ as a supplement. No reports have linked Vitamin B$_{12}$ with pregnancy complications. Vitamin B$_{12}$ has been assigned a risk factor category of A in recommended doses and a risk factor category of C in doses above the RDA (*see* Appendix 1).

THE BOTTOM LINE: The RDA of Vitamin B$_{12}$ is safe during pregnancy.

Vitamin C

Vitamin C, or ascorbic acid, is a water-soluble vitamin. Vitamin C is important for tissue repair and collagen formation. Vitamin C can be found in citrus fruits, tomatoes, and red peppers. The recommended daily allowance (RDA) for pregnancy is 70 milligrams.

CONCERNS: Mild to moderate Vitamin C excess or deficiency does not appear to cause any pregnancy complications. Vitamin C has been assigned a risk factor category of A in recommended doses and a risk factor category of C in doses above the RDA (*see* Appendix 1).

THE BOTTOM LINE: The RDA of Vitamin C is safe in pregnancy.

Vitamin D

Vitamin D is a fat-soluble vitamin. Vitamin D aids in the growth and maintenance of healthy bones. Vitamin D can be found in fortified dairy products and fish oils (*see* Fish oil) and can be obtained through exposure to the sun. The recommended daily allowance in pregnancy (RDA) is 400 international units.

CONCERNS: Excessive amounts of Vitamin D from supplements can be toxic in humans, causing bone loss and heart rate abnormalities. Vitamin D has a risk factor category of A in recommended doses and a risk factor category of D in doses above the RDA (*see* Appendix 1).

THE BOTTOM LINE: The RDA of Vitamin D is safe during pregnancy. Larger doses may be toxic and additional supplementation is not advised.

Vitamin E

Vitamin E is a fat-soluble vitamin. Its exact role in keeping the body healthy is not known. Vitamin E can be obtained from fats, oils, meats, fish, legumes, nuts, and soy. The recommended daily allowance (RDA) for Vitamin E in pregnancy is 10 milligrams.

CONCERNS: Recent studies have shown that high does of Vitamin E supplementation can cause an increased risk of death.

Vitamin E has a risk factor category of A in recommended doses and a risk factor category of C in doses above the RDA (*see* Appendix 1).

THE BOTTOM LINE: The RDA of Vitamin E is safe during pregnancy.

Vitamin K

Vitamin K is a fat-soluble vitamin that plays a role in the normal clotting of blood and in bone health. Vitamin K is found in soybean oil and dark leafy green vegetables. The recommended daily allowance (RDA) of Vitamin K during pregnancy is 75 micrograms.

CONCERNS: When taken in large doses at the end of the pregnancy, Vitamin K can cause some toxicity in the newborn.

THE BOTTOM LINE: The RDA of Vitamin K is safe during pregnancy.

Vitamins, multiple *See* Multivitamins.

Walking ✓

The American College of Obstetrics and Gynecology encourages most pregnant women to exercise for 30 minutes a day on most days. Walking is a great exercise (*see* Exercise) that requires very little equipment or training.

CONCERNS: Some women who are at risk of preterm labor are advised to limit their physical activity, including walking. This recommendation is directed only to women who have certain high-risk pregnancies. For everyone else, walking appears to be a safe and healthy form of exercise throughout pregnancy.

THE BOTTOM LINE: Walking is a safe, easy, and healthy form of exercise throughout pregnancy.

Water parks ⚠

Water parks offer many water activities, including pools, water slides, and lazy rivers.

CONCERNS: Water slides can generate high speeds and cause your abdomen to bump against slide edges (*see* Amusement park rides). The theoretical concern with these rides is the sudden starts and stops, which may be associated with placental abruption (premature separation of the placenta from the uterus). The jarring force from even slow automobile accidents has been known to cause placental abruption and other complications for pregnant women even when the trauma is not directly to the uterus.

Most water parks have water treated with chlorine (*see* Chlorine; Pools). The effects of chlorine and its metabolites during pregnancy are being investigated.

THE BOTTOM LINE: Consider avoiding activities in water parks that involve high speed, the possibility of abdominal trauma, and high chlorine levels. Use sunscreen to prevent the risks of sun damage (*see* Sun exposure).

Wellbutrin® ⚠

Wellbutrin® is a brand name for bupropion (*see* Psychiatric medications).

White tea *See* Tea. ⚠

Wine 🚫

Wine is a beverage made from fermented grapes (*see* Alcoholic beverages).

X rays ⚠

The term *X rays* is used to describe diagnostic radiologic studies using radiation. These studies include X rays, gastrointestinal (GI) series, and computed tomography (CT) scans.

CONCERNS: The type of radiation used in diagnostic radiologic studies is known to be teratogenic (causing birth defects) in high doses. However, studies that use less than 5 rads (a measure of radiation) are not thought to be harmful to the fetus. Most routine studies use very little radiation. For example, a chest X ray delivers 8 millirads of radiation.

THE BOTTOM LINE: Although large amounts of radiation can be harmful to a developing fetus, it is known that less than 5 rads is not dangerous. If you require an X ray during pregnancy, make sure the radiologist knows that you are pregnant so that proper precautions, such as abdominal shielding, can be taken to minimize your exposure. Avoid unnecessary X rays until after pregnancy. Avoid routine radiological studies such as mammograms or dental X rays until after pregnancy.

Xanax® 🚫

Xanax® is a brand name for alprazolam (*see* Psychiatric medications).

Yeast infection medication *See* Antifungal medications, oral and ☑️
topical; Diflucan; Fluconazole, Terconazole.

Yoga ☑️

Yoga is a form of exercise (*see* Exercise) involving a series of postures that
promote flexibility and strength. It is thought that yoga helps reduce
stress (*see* Stress), anxiety, and fear.

CONCERNS: Yoga instructors often offer some advice to those practic-
ing yoga while pregnant, including avoiding prolonged poses on the
back, as the weight of the fetus pressing against the aorta (a major artery) can restrict the blood flow to the lower body, including the uterus.
If you feel dizzy or light-headed while on your back, immediately bend
your knees and slowly roll over to your side. Avoid poses that stretch the
muscles too much, particularly the abdominal muscles. During pregnancy the amount of the hormone relaxin increases in the blood. Relaxin
is a hormone produced by the reproductive tract during pregnancy. Its
main role is to inhibit uterine contractions, soften the cervix, and dilate
blood vessels. Relaxin also works on other tissues such as ligaments and
can make it easier to strain muscles and ligaments while exercising.
Avoid all postures that put pressure on your abdomen, especially forward
folds, twists, and belly-down postures. Modify forward-folding poses
with the legs apart so the belly comes between the legs, and bend from
the hips, not the back. Modify the position of the legs in twists so the

legs do not press against the belly, and twist more from the shoulders and back. Listen carefully to your body. If you feel any discomfort, stop. You will probably need to adapt most postures to your body's physical changes. You may wish to restrict yourself to classes specifically labeled prenatal. Also use caution when doing Bikram (hot) yoga, as you can become dehydrated and light-headed. It is unknown whether Bikram yoga can raise your core body temperature, which is associated with certain birth defects.

THE BOTTOM LINE: With certain precautions, yoga is safe and beneficial during pregnancy.

Yogurt

Yogurt is a food made from milk that is fermented and coagulated by bacteria. Yogurt may be served plain or flavored with fruit and other ingredients. Some yogurt contains active live bacterial cultures, which are felt to aid in digestion (*see* Acidophilus; Probiotics).

CONCERNS: Yogurt contains calcium, protein, and potentially beneficial bacteria. Calcium requirements increase during pregnancy (*see* Calcium), and yogurt is a good way to meet some of these requirements. Avoid yogurt with artificial saccharin (*see* Artificial sweeteners; Saccharin).

THE BOTTOM LINE: It is safe and healthy to eat yogurt during pregnancy.

Zicam® ☑

Zicam® is the brand name for a variety of cold, allergy, and sinus remedies that are in the form of a nasal spray. They all contain zinc gluconate
(*see* Zinc), which is thought to prevent and/or shorten the duration of the
common cold.

CONCERNS: The main concern over the use of Zicam® is that there is little information about its effects on pregnancy. Using Zicam® may result
in ingesting more zinc than the Recommended Daily Allowance (RDA) of
zinc for pregnancy.

In 2007 Zicam® reached a settlement with consumers who alleged
that use of Zicam® products affected their sense of smell.

This product is considered a food supplement and it is not regulated
by the U.S. Food and Drug Administration (FDA). Thus there is no guarantee of the strength, purity, or safety of this product. You should inform
your health care provider if you are taking any nutritional supplements.

THE BOTTOM LINE: Although Zicam® is probably safe in pregnancy,
there is little information about is use during pregnancy to support or
discourage its use.

Zinc ☑

Zinc is an essential mineral that may help the immune system function
properly. Zinc requirements increase during pregnancy, and the recommended daily allowance (RDA) of zinc during pregnancy is 11 milligrams

(mg) per day. Zinc can be obtained from meat, fortified cereals, shellfish (*see* Shellfish), poultry, beans, nuts, and dairy products, and is also found in multivitamins (*see* Multivitamins). Zinc deficiency in the United States is rare except in people with digestive disorders or alcoholism.

CONCERNS: Zinc deficiency in laboratory animals has been associated with fetal growth retardation (low birth weight) and fetal abnormalities. However, a large study examining women's zinc levels and pregnancy outcomes failed to show any association between zinc levels and pregnancy complications. The National Academy of Sciences recommends no more than 40 mg a day of zinc from all sources.

THE BOTTOM LINE: Zinc deficiency is rare in the United States due to its presence in a variety of foods. Multivitamins contain zinc, and additional supplements are not needed.

Zithromax®

Zithromax® is the brand name for azithromycin (*see* Azithromycin; Antibiotics, oral).

Zoloft®

Zoloft® is a brand name for sertraline (*see* Psychiatric medications).

Zyrtec®

Zyrtec® is a brand name of cetrizine (*see* Allergy medications; Cetrizine).

FOOD AND DRUG ADMINISTRATION
RISK FACTOR CATEGORIES

CATEGORY	DESCRIPTION
A	Adequate, well-controlled studies in pregnant women have not shown an increased risk of fetal abnormalities.
B	Animal studies have revealed no evidence of harm to the fetus; however, there are no adequate well-controlled studies in pregnant women.
	or
	Animal studies have shown an adverse effect, but adequate and well-controlled studies in pregnant women have failed to demonstrate a risk to the fetus.
C	Animal studies have shown an adverse effect, and there are no adequate and well-controlled studies in pregnant women.
	or
	No animal studies have been conducted, and there are no adequate and well-controlled studies in pregnant women.
D	Studies, adequate well-controlled or observational, in pregnant women have demonstrated a risk to the fetus. However, the benefits of therapy may outweigh the potential risk.

X   Studies, adequate well-controlled or observational, in animals or pregnant women have demonstrated positive evidence of fetal abnormalities. The use of this product is contraindicated in women who are or may become pregnant.

www.acog.org

The American College of Obstetrics and Gynecology (ACOG) Web site. ACOG works to maintain standards for women's health, offers postgraduate training to physicians, and provides for patient education and advocacy. Search for information on women's health and pregnancy. Search for board-certified/board-eligible physicians in your area.

www.ahealthyme.com

The Healthy Me Web site produced by the *Consumer Health Interactive* editorial team. Search for articles and information relating to women's health and health issues during pregnancy.

www.babycenter.com

The Baby Center Web site. Their editorial team has worked at major magazines, such as *Parenting*, *Parents*, and *Health*. Articles are thoroughly researched and fact-checked. Search for information on women's health and pregnancy.

www.cdc.gov

The Centers for Disease Control and Prevention (CDC) Web site. This federal agency works to improve the health of people. Search for information about specific diseases, treatments, and vaccinations.

www.cpsc.gov

The U.S. Consumer Product Safety Commission Web site. This independent federal regulatory agency works to protect the public from products that pose a fire, electrical, chemical, or mechanical hazard or can injure children. Search for articles and information relating to product safety news and product recalls.

www.epa.gov

The Environmental Protection Agency (EPA) Web site. The EPA, headed by the administrator who is appointed by the president of the United States, works to improve the health of people and the environment. Search for information on environmental hazards.

www.fda.gov

The U.S. Food and Drug Administration (FDA) Web site. According to its literature, the FDA is a "governmental agency that is responsible for protecting the public health by assuring the safety, efficacy, and security of human and veterinary drugs, biological products, medical devices, our nation's food supply, cosmetics, and products that emit radiation. The FDA is also responsible for advancing the public health by helping to speed innovations that make medicines and foods more effective, safer, and more affordable; and helping the public get the accurate, science-based information they need to use medicines and foods to improve their health." Search here for information on drugs, food safety, and medical devices.

www.intelihealth.com

This Web site contains medical information written by the Natural Standard and the Harvard Medical School. Use this Web site to search for issues relating to women's health and pregnancy.

www.mayoclinic.com

The Mayo Clinic Web site. Medical content is created by the Mayo Clinic. Search for information on women's health and pregnancy.

www.modimes.org

The March of Dimes Web site. Search here for information on women's health, pregnancy, and birth defects.

www.motherisk.org

The Motherisk Web site. The Motherisk Team is "an experienced, multi-disciplinary group of scientists and clinicians with expertise in areas such as addiction research, clinical pharmacology, genetics, nutrition, obstetrics, preventive medicine and psychology." All are affiliated with the University of Toronto. Search here for information about exposure to drugs and toxins.

www.nih.gov

The National Institutes of Health (NIH) Web site. The NIH, an agency under the U.S. Department of Health and Human Services, is the steward of medical and behavioral research for the nation. Search for information on a variety of health concerns.

www.osha.gov

The United States Department of Labor Occupational Safety and Health Administration (OSHA) Web site. OSHA's mission is "to assure the safety and health of America's workers by setting and enforcing standards; providing training, outreach, and education; establishing partnerships; and encouraging continual improvement in workplace safety and health." Search here for information about hazards in the workplace.

www.OTISpregnancy.org

The Organization of Teratology Information Services (OTIS) Web site. Teratology Information Services (TIS) are comprehensive and multidisciplinary resources for medical consultation on prenatal exposures. TIS interpret information regarding known and potential reproductive risks into risk assessments that are communicated to individuals of reproductive age and health care providers.

www.perinatology.com

Perinatology.com is maintained by the San Gabriel Valley Perinatal Medical Group, under license from Focus Information Technology, as an educational resource for perinatologists, referring physicians, and genetic counselors. Information on the site has been written by perinatologists and genetic counselors. There are links to various sites. Use this site to search for information about exposure to drugs and toxins.

www.pregnancytoday.com

The Pregnancy Today Web site, sponsored by iParenting Media, a media company focused on parents. Search for information relating to women's health and pregnancy.

www.pubmed.net

A Web site sponsored by the National Institutes of Health and used by researchers and physicians to search for abstracts and scientific articles.

www.safefetus.com

A Web site maintained by physicians and pharmacists to provide information on the effects of drugs during pregnancy and breastfeeding. Search for common drugs and their risk factor categories.

toxnet.nlm.nih.gov/cgi-bin/sis/htmlgen?TOXLINE

A search engine for scientific studies on potentially toxic substances set up by the National Institutes of Health's National Library of Medicine Web site. Search for scientific articles on specific drugs, chemicals, and toxins.

http://householdproducts.nlm.nih.gov

A search engine set up by the National Institutes of Health's National Library of Medicine Web site. Search for household products to learn of any potential effects.

This appendix briefly describes some illnesses mentioned in the text as well as a few others that you might come across in your reading.

Aflatoxicosis

Aflatoxicosis is a condition that results from poisoning due to ingestion of aflatoxins in contaminated food. Cases of food contaminated with aflatoxins have been seen with tree nuts, peanuts, and other oil seeds, including corn and cottonseed. Aflatoxicosis in humans is rare, but has been reported. Aflatoxins may be carcinogenic (cancer causing) in humans.

Amebiasis

Amebiasis is caused by the parasite *Entamoeba histolytica*. This parasite can be acquired through the ingestion of contaminated water or food. It is most common in developing countries that have poor sanitation. Only 10 percent of people infected with this parasite will have any symptoms. Symptoms include loose stools and stomach pains. This parasite can spread to the liver, brain, and lungs rarely. Diagnosis is made by having your stool examined and it can be treated with antibiotics. You can reduce your risk of acquiring this parasite by boiling water for one minute, avoiding food sold from street vendors, avoiding unpasteurized dairy products, and peeling fruits and vegetables prior to eating when traveling to areas with poor sanitation.

Botulism

Botulism is caused by a group of bacteria called *Clostridium botulinum*. These bacteria are found in soil. Botulism is most common in young children, but it can also affect adults, most commonly as a result of improper home canning. *Botulinum* spores can be found in honey, and *botulinum* toxin is used in anti-wrinkle injections such as Botox®.

Chicken pox *See* **Varicella disease.**

Chlamydia

Chlamydia is caused by the bacterium *Chlamydia trachomatis*, which requires cells to grow. It is one of the most common sexually transmitted infections in the United States. Chlamydia can affect both men and women and can be spread through sexual contact and through the birth canal to a newborn. Because many women have chlamydial infections without symptoms, women are routinely screened for the disease during pregnancy. Some women will have symptoms including vaginal discharge, bleeding, and pain. Chlamydia can be treated with antibiotics.

Cholera

Cholera is a disease caused by the bacterium *Vibrio cholerae*. Symptoms include diarrhea, vomiting, and leg cramps. The illness can be mild or severe. Cholera is rare in industrialized countries due to good sanitation, but still exists in India and sub-Saharan Africa. The bacteria can be spread through contaminated water and food.

Cryptospiridosis

Intestinal cryptospiridosis is caused by the *Cryptosporidium parvum* protozoan. Its symptoms include watery diarrhea, but the disease may also be asymptomatic. The protozoa can also affect the respiratory system, causing cough and fever. Outbreaks are associated with child care centers, contaminated water supplies, and uncooked vegetables grown in contaminated fertilizer.

Cytomegalovirus infection

Cytomegalovirus (CMV) is a virus that is universally present. The Centers for Disease Control and Prevention estimates that in the United States, 50 to 85 percent of adults are infected by CMV by age 40. CMV infection is usually not dangerous unless you are in an immunocompromised state or are pregnant. CMV infection during pregnancy can put the fetus at risk for congenital CMV disease, which can lead to hearing loss, vision impairment, and varying degrees of mental retardation. Immunity to CMV can be determined by a blood test.

Diphtheria

Diphtheria is caused by the bacterium *Corynebacterium diphtheriae*, which produces a poison that enters the bloodstream. Symptoms include sore throat, mild fever, and swollen lymph nodes. Diphtheria is rare in the United States due to routine immunization during childhood.

E. coli infection

E. coli infection is caused by a bacterium called *Escherichia coli*. Most strains of *E. coli* are safe, and many exist in our intestines and act to help make some vitamins, such as Vitamin K. However, some strains can cause disease. *E. coli* O157:H7 can cause diarrhea and potentially be life threatening. You can ingest this bacterium from contaminated meat (improperly cooked hamburger meat has been implicated), unpasteurized juices, and vegetables.

German measles *See* Rubella.

Giardiasis

Giardiasis is caused by a protozoan named *Giardia lamblia*. It is the most frequent cause of nonbacterial diarrhea in North America. The symptoms include diarrhea, weight loss, and malabsorption (inability to absorb nutrients from the intestines). Infected people may be asymptomatic. According to the Centers for Disease Control and Prevention, approximately 2 percent of the population in the United States has had giardiasis. *Giardia* can be acquired from contaminated water or raw vegetables or may be sexually transmitted, and is common in child day care centers in which diapering is done. Giardiasis can be treated with the antibiotic metronidazole (Flagyl®).

Hepatitis A

Hepatitis A is caused by the hepatitis A virus (HAV). It causes inflammation of the liver and liver disease. Symptoms include jaundice (yellow color of skin), fatigue, abdominal pain, nausea, diarrhea, and fever. It is transmitted through a person's infected stool or through food contaminated with the HAV. Water, shellfish, and salads are the most common foods that have been implicated in outbreaks. A vaccination is available.

Hepatitis B

Hepatitis B is caused by the hepatitis B virus (HBV). It can cause lifelong infection, scarring of the liver, and death. Symptoms include jaundice (yellow color of the skin), fatigue, abdominal pain, nausea, vomiting, and joint pain. It is spread through infected body fluids. A vaccine is available. All pregnant women are tested for hepatitis B in order to provide treatment to the infant after birth.

Hepatitis C

Hepatitis C is caused by the hepatitis C virus. It is spread through contact with infected blood. People at risk of acquiring this virus include people who receive blood transfusions or blood products, intravenous drug users, and dialysis patients. There is no vaccination available for this virus. There is a 4 percent risk of transmitting the virus during pregnancy. The Centers for Disease Control and Prevention estimates that 3.0 million (1.8 percent) Americans have been infected with the hepatitis C virus.

HIV/AIDs

HIV/AIDs is caused by the human immunodeficiency virus. This virus can be found in infected blood, semen, breast milk, and vaginal secretions. The virus can be transmitted during pregnancy, but the risk of transmission has been dramatically decreased with proper treatment during pregnancy. Because of this, all women should be screened for HIV/AIDs during pregnancy. The Centers for Disease Control and Prevention estimates that at the end of 2003, 1,039,000 to 1,185,000 persons in the United States had HIV/AIDs. They also estimate that 24 to 27 percent of persons having HIV/AIDs do not know that they are infected with the virus.

Influenza

Influenza, also known as the flu, is a viral illness characterized by fever, muscle aches, sore throat, and cough. The flu is spread through infected respiratory droplets. The flu may be more severe in pregnant women, and some research has shown an association between influenza during pregnancy and the development of schizophrenia in the child. As a result, the Centers for Disease Control and Prevention recommends that all pregnant women receive a flu vaccine regardless of trimester.

Legionnaire's disease

Legionnaire's disease is caused by the bacterium *Legionella pneumophila*. The disease is characterized by pneumonia. The Centers for Disease Control and Prevention estimates that 8,000 to 18,000 people acquire Legionnaire's disease in the United States each year. A milder form of the disease caused by the same organism is known as Pontiac fever. Pontiac fever is characterized by fever and muscle aches, but not pneumonia.

Listeriosis

Listeriosis is an illness caused by the bacterium *Listeria monocytogenes*. Symptoms include fever, muscle aches, and gastrointestinal symptoms. Infection can complicate pregnancy by causing stillbirth, preterm labor, or infection of the newborn. Pregnant women are 20 times more likely to get listeriosis than other healthy adults. According to the Centers for Disease Control and Prevention, 2,500 people get listeriosis per year, and one-third of these cases occur in pregnant women. Listeria can contaminate raw fruits, vegetables, meat, unpasteurized dairy products, and soft cheese.

Lyme disease

Lyme disease is caused by the bacterium *Borrelia burgdorferi*, which is transmitted by the bite of an infected deer tick. Acute symptoms include fever, skin rash, joint inflammation, and flu-like effects. Chronic infection can lead to more serious problems, including heart, joint, and neurological symptoms. It is unclear how Lyme disease affects pregnancy. The disease is best treated in the acute stage; take proper precautions against being bitten if you live in an area in which the disease is present.

Malaria

Malaria is caused by a parasite that enters your body after a bite from an infected mosquito. After the parasite enters the bloodstream, it migrates to the liver, where it matures and then reenters the bloodstream to infect the red blood cells. Symptoms of malaria include fever, muscle aches, chills, nausea, and vomiting. Malaria can be transmitted across the placenta to infect the fetus.

Measles

Measles, also known as rubeola, is caused by a virus. The incidence of measles in the United States is rare, due to routine childhood immunization. Symptoms include fever, cough, rash, and spots in the mouth. The disease is spread in infected respiratory droplets through sneezing. The vaccination for measles should not be given to pregnant women.

Mumps

Mumps is a viral infection caused by a paramyxovirus. It is not very common in the United States due to routine vaccination during childhood. Symptoms include swollen glands, fever, weakness, pain with swallowing, and tenderness of the testicles. The disease can be spread by contact with infected saliva and with infected respiratory droplets through sneezing. Women who are pregnant are at an increased risk for miscarriage if they receive the vaccine during the first trimester of pregnancy. The vaccination for mumps should not be given to pregnant women.

Perfringens food poisoning

The bacterium *Clostridium perfringens* can cause perfringens food poisoning. The bacteria release a toxin, which is the cause of the illness. Symptoms include diarrhea and abdominal cramps. In most cases, the cause of the illness is improper cooling of prepared foods. Small numbers of organisms present in food after cooking can multiply to food poisoning levels during food cooldown and storage. Meats and gravies are frequently implicated. To avoid this problem, store foods in small containers so they cool down more quickly and use caution when eating foods left on low heat, such as on steamer tables.

Plague

Plague is a disease caused by the bacterium *Yersinia pestis*. It is generally transmitted after being bitten by an infected rodent flea. Rats, rabbits, and prairie dogs can be affected. Plague is not common in the United States today, but outbreaks can occur. Symptoms include pneumonia, coughing, fever, muscle aches, headache, and swollen lymph nodes. Once infected, humans can spread the disease to others by coughing. This disease can be treated with antibiotics.

Pneumococcal pneumonia

Pneumococcal pneumonia and meningitis is caused by the bacterium *Streptococcus pneumoniae*. The disease affects the elderly and the immunocompromised most often. Currently a vaccine is available, but it generally should not be given to pregnant women.

Poliomyelitis

Poliomyelitis (polio) is caused by a virus called poliovirus. Symptoms include fever, headache, sore throat, neck stiffness, back pain, muscle pains, and paralysis. There are varying degrees of infection. Because most children in this country are routinely vaccinated against this virus, polio is rare in the United States. Polio still exists in several places around the world.

Pseudomonas infection

Pseudomonas infection is caused by the bacterium *Pseudomonas aeruginosa*. Pseudomonas can cause a wide range of infections, including pneumonia, urinary tract infections (UTIs), bone infections, and endocarditis (infection of the valves of the heart). The bacteria are widespread and will only infect tissues that are compromised or patients who are immunocompromised. This infection can be treated with antibiotics.

Rabies

Rabies is caused by the rabies virus. You can contract rabies after being bitten by an infected animal. Symptoms include fever, headache, malaise, anxiety, insomnia, and confusion. Wild carnivores and bats are the most commonly affected animals today. A vaccine can be administered either after you have been exposed to rabies or to people who are at high risk of acquiring rabies.

Rocky Mountain spotted fever

Rocky Mountain spotted fever is caused by the *Rickettsia rickettsii* bacterium. The disease is spread through the bite of an infected tick. Symptoms include fever, headache, muscle pain, and rash. The disease can also be spread if you crush a tick and you have any scrapes on your hand through which the disease can enter your body. The disease is treated with the antibiotic tetracycline or doxycycline, both of which should not be taken during pregnancy.

Rubella

Rubella, also known as German measles, is caused by the rubella virus. Rubella is rare in the United States, due to routine childhood vaccination. Symptoms include fever, swollen lymph nodes, and rash. Rubella is dangerous during pregnancy, as the virus can cross the placenta and infect the baby, causing congenital rubella syndrome. All pregnant women are screened for immunity to rubella and if nonimmune are vaccinated after delivery.

Rubeolla *See* Measles.

Salmonellosis

Salmonellosis is caused by a group of bacteria called *Salmonella*. Salmonellosis is characterized by a gastrointestinal illness including diarrhea, abdominal cramps, and fever. Salmonellosis can be acquired from infected raw poultry, eggs, and raw vegetables. Reptiles are also known to carry *Salmonella*. *Salmonella* can be spread through improper hand washing. The Centers for Disease Control and Prevention estimates that 40,000 cases of salmonellosis are reported every year.

Staphylococcus food poisoning

Staphylococcal food poisoning is caused by the bacterium *Staphylococcus aureus*. These bacteria are everywhere, but can multiply in foods under the right conditions (below 140°F and above 45°F) and produce an endotoxin that causes disease. Symptoms include nausea, vomiting, abdominal cramping, and headache. Foods that are frequently incriminated in staphylococcal food poisoning include meat, poultry, eggs, and diary products. Foods that are kept at slightly elevated temperatures and are handled a lot during the preparation are often affected. These include salads, such as tuna, egg, chicken, pasta, and potato, as well as baked goods with dairy fillings, such as éclairs. The disease is usually self-limiting and death is rare.

Tapeworms

Tapeworms are parasitic flatworms that spend part of their life cycle in the intestines of humans or animals. The most common tapeworm in the United States is the beef tapeworm (*Taenia saginata*). There is also a pork tapeworm (*Taenia solium*) and a fish tapeworm (*Diphyllobothrium latum*). Infestation is usually without symptoms, but there may be abdominal discomfort, diarrhea, constipation, or weight loss. Tapeworms are killed during proper cooking of food. Quinacrine hydrochloride or niclosamide is given to treat the disease.

Toxoplasmosis

Toxoplasmosis is caused by a parasite, *Toxoplasmosis gondii*. Toxoplasmosis is common in the United States. The Centers for Disease Control and Prevention estimates that more than 60 million people in the country may be infected with this parasite. It usually causes only a mild disease with symptoms similar to the flu, including muscle aches and swollen lymph nodes. However, it can be more dangerous if you are pregnant, as it can cross the placenta and infect the baby. Toxoplasmosis can be acquired through eating contaminated meat, vegetables, and water. It can also be acquired from accidentally ingesting contaminated cat feces. Treatment is available, but not always necessary, in mild cases. Although the parasite remains within your body, most people develop immunity to this disease.

Trichinosis

Trichinosis is caused by a roundworm called *Trichinella spiralis*. It can be acquired by eating raw or undercooked meat, most commonly pork. There are approximately 40 cases per year in the United States. Symptoms of infection include abdominal pain, diarrhea, fever, and muscle aches. To prevent this illness, eat only well-done pork. Curing, smoking, or salting pork does not always eliminate this parasite.

Trichomoniasis

Trichomoniasis is caused by a parasite called *Trichomonas vaginalis*. Vaginal infection is often characterized by discharge, odor, and burning with urination, but may be asymptomatic. Diagnosis is made by looking for the organism under a microscope after obtaining a vaginal smear. Infection can be treated with the antibiotic metronidazole. Infection during pregnancy has been associated with an increased risk of premature rupture of membranes and preterm labor.

Tuberculosis

Tuberculosis is caused by *Mycobacterium tuberculosis*. Infection with tuberculosis can be asymptomatic or can be characterized by cough, fever, and night sweats. During pregnancy, tuberculosis is generally treated with the drug isoniazid. Transmission to the fetus is rare, but has been known to complicate pregnancy.

Typhoid fever

Typhoid fever is caused by the bacterium *Salmonella typhi*. The Centers for Disease Control and Prevention estimates that there are 400 cases per year in the United States; most are acquired during international travel. You can get typhoid fever from food or water handled by an infected person or from contaminated water. Travel to Asia, Africa, and Latin America will put you at risk for acquiring this disease. Symptoms include high fever, stomach pains, and headache. A vaccination is available.

Varicella disease

Varicella disease is more commonly known as chicken pox or zoster. Varicella is caused by a virus called the varicella-zoster virus. Symptoms include a blisterlike rash, itching, fever, and malaise. Chicken pox is spread from person to person through coughing and sneezing. A vaccination is available against chicken pox. Chicken pox can be more dangerous during pregnancy, as the symptoms can be more severe and the virus can be transmitted to the fetus. Once you have had chicken pox, you acquire immunity; it is rare to get chicken pox again.

Waterborne diseases

Waterborne diseases include any disease that can be acquired through contaminated water. Some of these include amebiasis, cholera, giardiasis, hepatitis A, and salmonellosis. These diseases are generally acquired from sewage-contaminated water. Please see individual diseases for details.

Yellow fever

Yellow fever is a mosquito-borne viral disease caused by the yellow fever virus. This disease occurs only in sub-Saharan Africa and tropical South America. Symptoms include fever, muscle aches, hepatitis, and hemorrhagic fever. A vaccination is available.

Zoonotic disease

The term *zoonotic disease* is used to describe disease that can be acquired from animals. Zoonotic diseases include toxoplasmosis and yellow fever. Please see individual diseases for details.

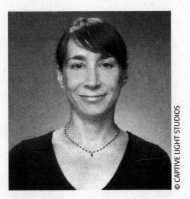

© CAPTIVE LIGHT STUDIOS

DR. ELISABETH ARON is an award-winning, board-certified obstetrician and gynecologist and a senior clinical instructor at the University of Colorado's Department of Obstetrics and Gynecology. She lives in Fort Collins, Colorado.